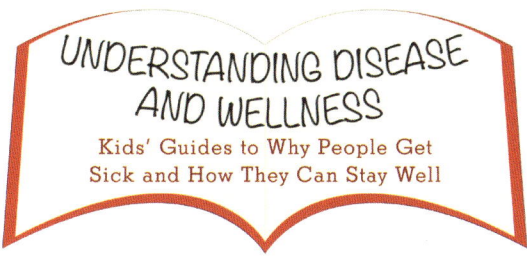

A KID'S GUIDE TO VIRUSES & BACTERIA

Rae Simons

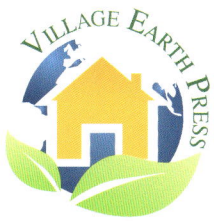

Series List

A Kid's Guide to a Healthier You
A Kid's Guide to AIDS and HIV
A Kid's Guide to Allergies
A Kid's Guide to Asthma
A Kid's Guide to Bugs and How They Can Make You Sick
A Kid's Guide to Cancer
A Kid's Guide to Diabetes
A Kid's Guide to Drugs and Alcohol
A Kid's Guide to Immunizations
A Kid's Guide to Malnutrition
A Kid's Guide to Obesity
A Kid's Guide to Pollution and How It Can Make You Sick
A Kid's Guide to Viruses and Bacteria

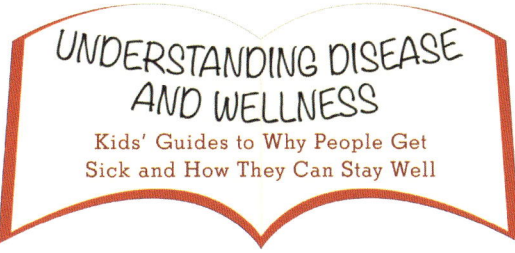

A KID'S GUIDE TO VIRUSES & BACTERIA

Rae Simons

Understanding Disease and Wellness:
Kids' Guides to Why People Get Sick and How They Can Stay Well
A KID'S GUIDE TO VIRUSES AND BACTERIA

Copyright © 2014 by Village Earth Press, a division of Harding House Publishing. All rights reserved. No part of this publication may be reproduced or transmitted in any form or by any means, electronic or mechanical, including photocopying, recording, taping, or any information storage and retrieval system, without permission from the publisher.

Village Earth Press
Vestal, New York 13850
www.villageearthpress.com

First Printing
9 8 7 6 5 4 3 2 1

Series ISBN: 978-1-62524-022-4
ISBN: 978-1-62524-033-0
ebook ISBN: 978-1-62524-055-2
Library of Congress Control Number: 2013911248

Author: Simons, Rae

Note: This book is a revised and updated edition of *Things You Can't See Can Make You Sick! Viruses & Bacteria* (ISBN: 978-1-934970-16-4), published in 2009 by Alpha House Publishing.

Introduction

According to a recent study reported in the Virginia Henderson International Nursing Library, kids worry about getting sick. They worry about AIDS and cancer, about allergies and the "super-germs" that resist medication. They know about these ills—but they don't always understand what causes them or how they can be prevented.

Unfortunately, most 9- to 11-year-olds, the study found, get their information about diseases like AIDS from friends and television; only 20 percent of the children interviewed based their understanding of illness on facts they had learned at school. Too often, kids believe urban legends, schoolyard folktales, and exaggerated movie plots. Oftentimes, misinformation like this only makes their worries worse. The January 2008 *Child Health News* reported that 55 percent of all children between 9 and 13 "worry almost all the time" about illness.

This series, **Understanding Disease and Wellness**, offers readers clear information on various illnesses and conditions, as well as the immunizations that can prevent many diseases. The books dispel the myths with clearly presented facts and colorful, accurate illustrations. Better yet, these books will help kids understand not only illness—but also what they can do to stay as healthy as possible.

—*Dr. Elise Berlan*

Just the Facts

- Germs are tiny creatures so small you can't see them without using a microscope. They can make humans sick.

- Germs are spread through our saliva, our breath, and our skin. We can also catch germs from the water we drink, the air we breathe, and some kinds of animals.

- Bacteria are the oldest life form on Earth. They come in 3 shapes: rods, balls, and spirals. Staph, strep, E. coli, and TB are all kinds of bacteria.

- Bacteria can be treated with antibiotics. However, so many people use antibiotics that many bacteria are starting to resist them.

- Viruses are even smaller than bacteria. They are not thought to be really alive. They need a host cell to reproduce or exist.

- The cold, pink eye, the flu, herpes, and HIV are all different kinds of viruses.

- There is no cure for viruses. Most of the time, doctors can only treat the symptoms, while your body fights the viruses. However, some vaccines can keep you from getting viruses.

- You can stay healthy by washing your hands, getting vaccines, and making sure you get enough sleep and eat a healthy diet.

What Are Germs?

You've probably heard someone say, "Don't touch that! It's germy." When people say this, they mean tiny, *microscopic* creatures are on whatever you're about to touch. These creatures are so small you can't see them—but if they get inside your body, they can make you sick. A cut in your skin is one way germs might get inside you. Or germs could be in something you eat or drink. Sometimes they're in the air, and you breathe them in. Germs are our tiniest enemies!

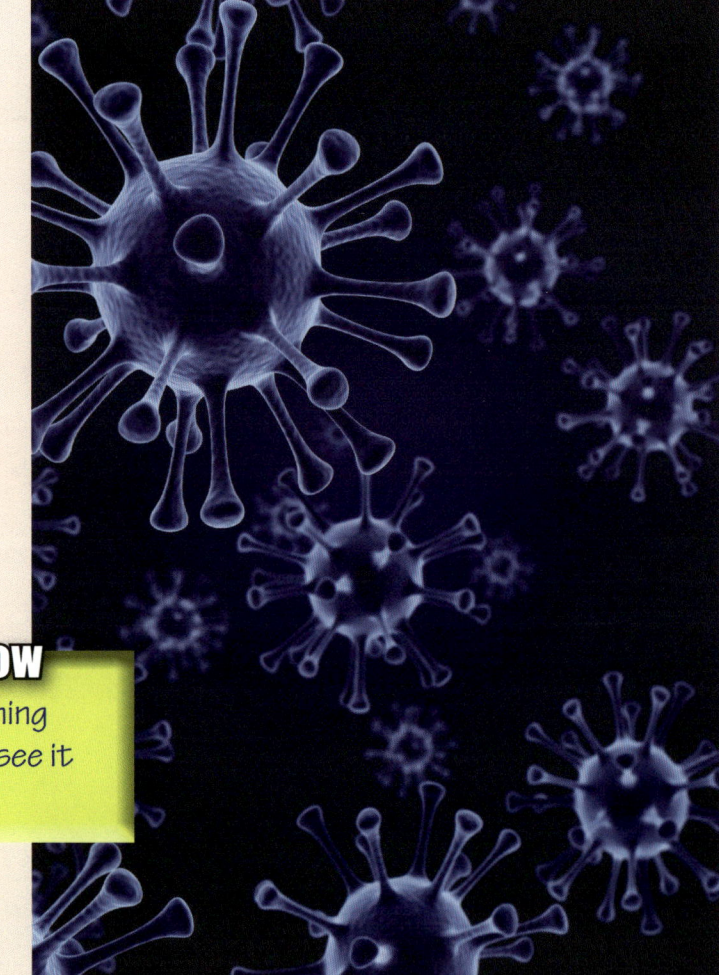

Words to Know

Microscopic: something so small you can only see it with a microscope.

Sometimes scientists use the word "microbes" to talk about germs. The most common microbes are bacteria and viruses. Both can make you sick, but each acts differently when it's inside your body.

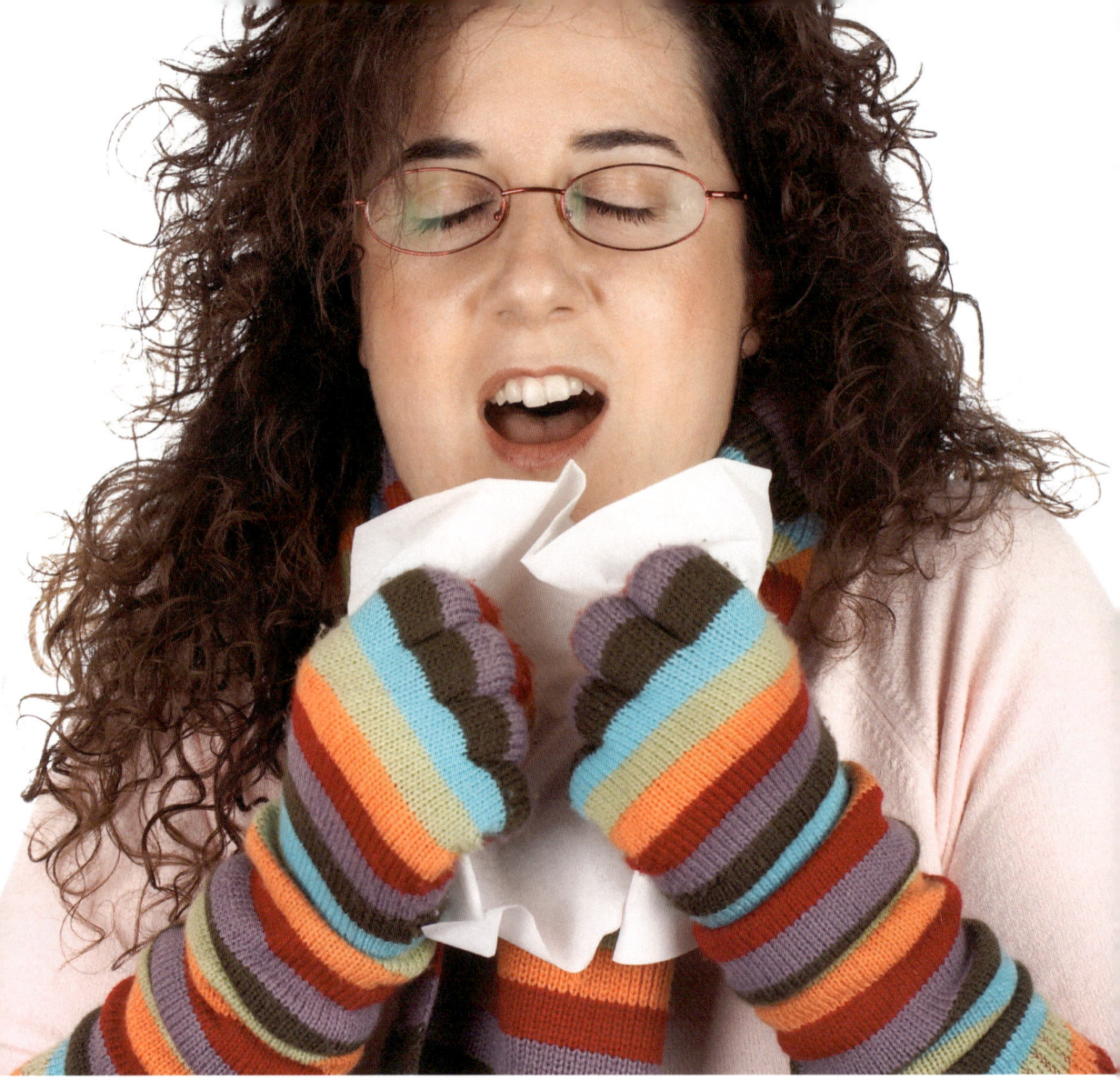

How Are Germs Spread?

Whenever someone sneezes, germs fly into the air. If the person sneezes into her hand or elbow, she catches them—but if she doesn't wash her hands, she will spread the germs to whatever and whomever she touches. We spread germs in our saliva, in our breath, and on our skin.

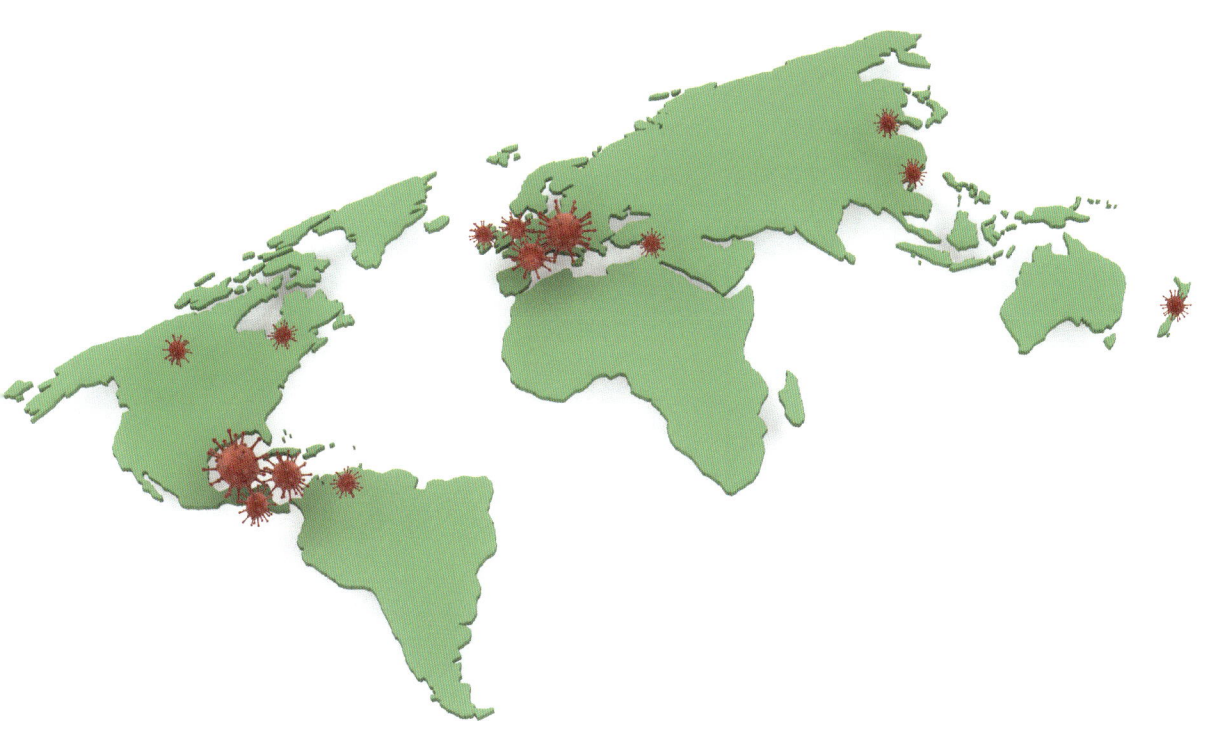

Some germs are more common in certain parts of the world than in others. For example, this map shows where the germ that causes swine flu is most likely to show up. Long ago, when people traveled less, each kind of germ was more likely to stay in one place. Now, however, it's fairly common for people to travel from place to place around the globe. This means diseases can spread more easily from one part of the world to another.

Germs are also spread in foods and in water. Some germs are carried by animals, including birds and insects.

What Are Bacteria?

Bacteria are one-celled *organisms* that come in three different shapes: rods (like the ones shown on these pages), balls, and spirals. They have been around for millions of years, since before the dinosaurs. In fact, they were probably the earliest form of life on Earth.

Bacteria live everywhere. They are in the air, in soil, and in water. They're in and on plants and animals—including you!

Words to Know

Organisms: living things that can function (eat, move, reproduce) independently (instead of being part of another animal or plant).

Atmosphere: the gases (the air) that surround our planet, allowing life to exist on Earth.

A single teaspoon of soil from your garden contains about a billion bacteria. Your mouth is home to more than five hundred different kinds of bacteria. Bacteria even live in places where nothing else can survive, like the boiling waters inside hot springs or in the bitter cold of the South Pole.

Although some bacteria can make you sick, most of these tiny creatures are actually very useful. Our world wouldn't be the same without them. They break down garbage, help our bodies make vitamins, and even help keep our *atmosphere* healthy.

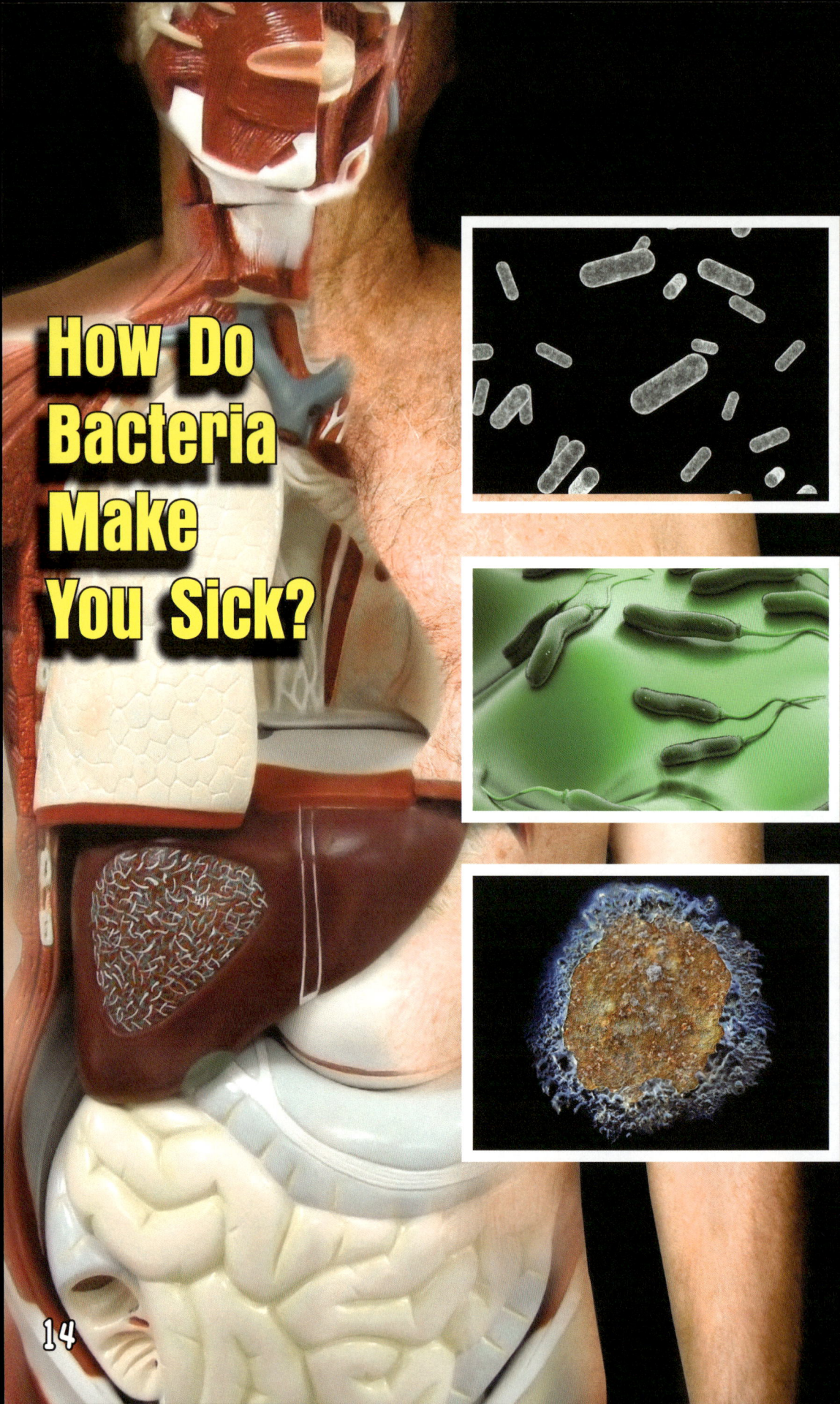

How Do Bacteria Make You Sick?

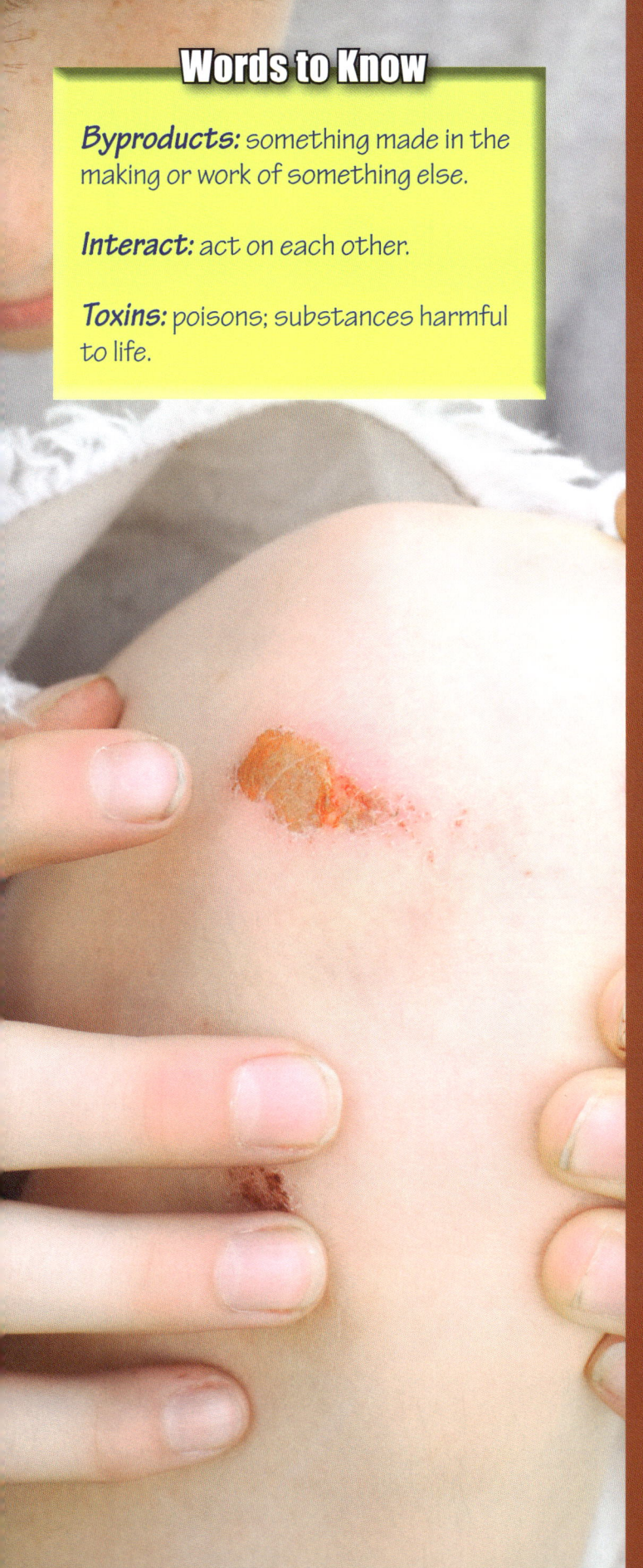

Words to Know

Byproducts: something made in the making or work of something else.

Interact: act on each other.

Toxins: poisons; substances harmful to life.

When some kinds of bacteria get inside your body, they produce chemicals as *byproducts* of the things they do to live. These chemicals then *interact* with your body's cells. They may make *toxins* that keep your body from doing its job in different ways.

The picture on the left page shows three different kinds of bacteria. If these bacteria get inside your body—for instance, through even a small scrape—they can make you sick in different ways.

15

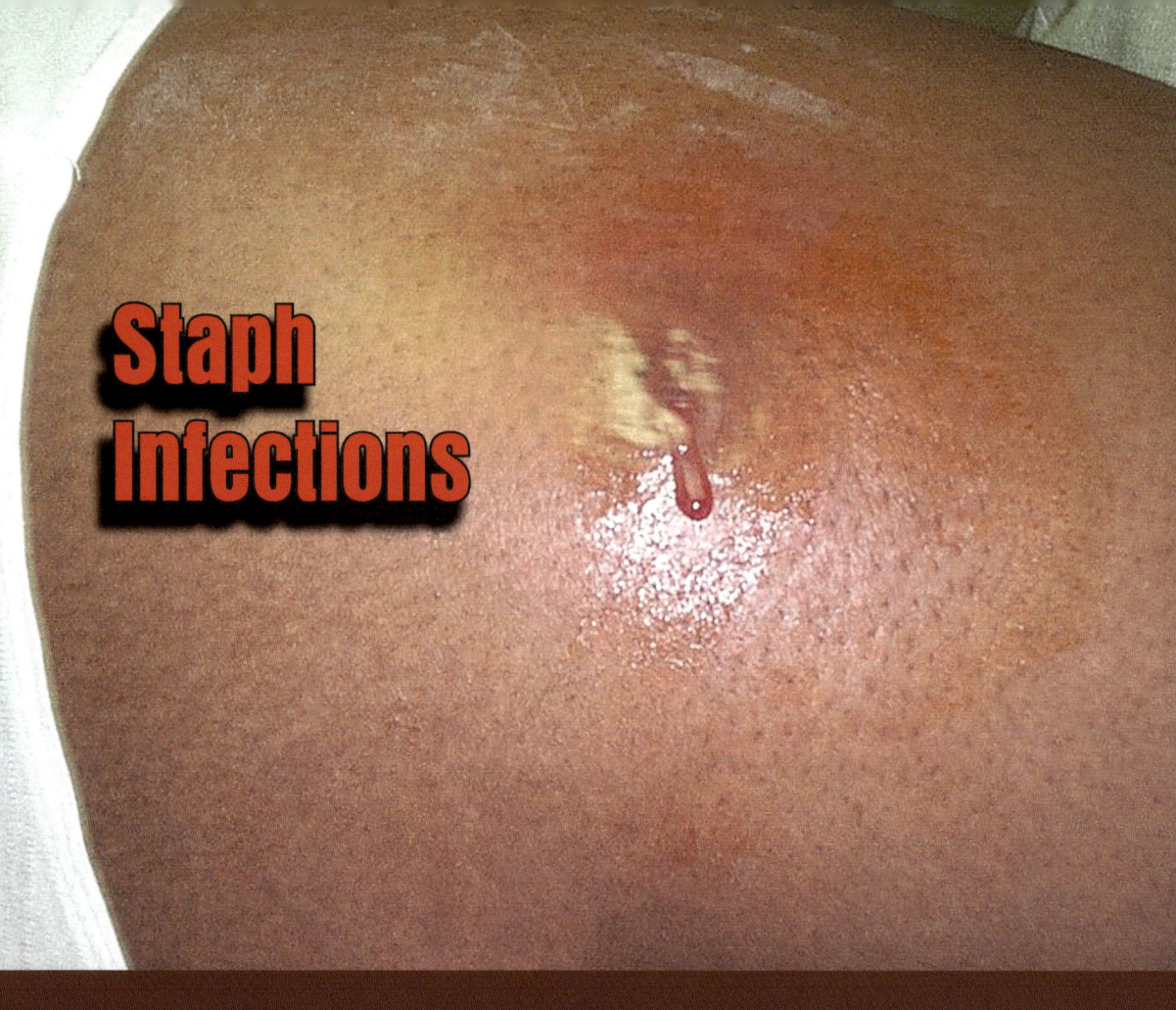

Staph Infections

Staph infections are one way bacteria can make you sick. "Staph" is short for *Staphylococcus aureus*. That's the scientific name for the bacteria shown in the picture above on the left. The name comes from two Greek words: *staphyle,* meaning a bunch of grapes, and *kokkos,* meaning berry. Scientists thought that under the microscope this bacteria looked like a bunch of grapes or little round berries.

This bacteria lives on your skin and in your nose much of the time. Usually, it doesn't make you sick. But when your skin is cut or broken (even if the cut is very tiny), staph bacteria can go inside your body. Then you may get sick. Staph bacteria can cause an infection in a sore like the one on the left page.

Staph bacteria can spread through the air too. It's often on doorknobs, tabletops, and other surfaces. People can also pass this bacteria from person to person when they touch each other. You can even carry staph bacteria with your fingers from one part of your body to another. Sometimes, staph can get inside your stomach and make you feel sick. Staph bacteria causes infections in other parts of your body as well. Swimmer's ear (that sore, itchy feeling you sometimes get in your ears after swimming), eye infections, and sore throats can all be caused by staph.

Good hand washing is the best way to keep from passing—and getting—staph infections. If you have a cut or a wound, be sure to keep it clean and covered. That way, staph bacteria can't get into it.

ASK THE DOCTOR

I have a sore spot on my eyelid. My mother says it's a stye, and that I got it from reading too much. Is that true?

Answer: No, eyestrain does not cause styes. A stye (also known as a hordeolum) is a staph infection in the eyelid. It makes glands at the base of the eyelash become swollen and sore. A warm washcloth can soothe styes and help them heal.

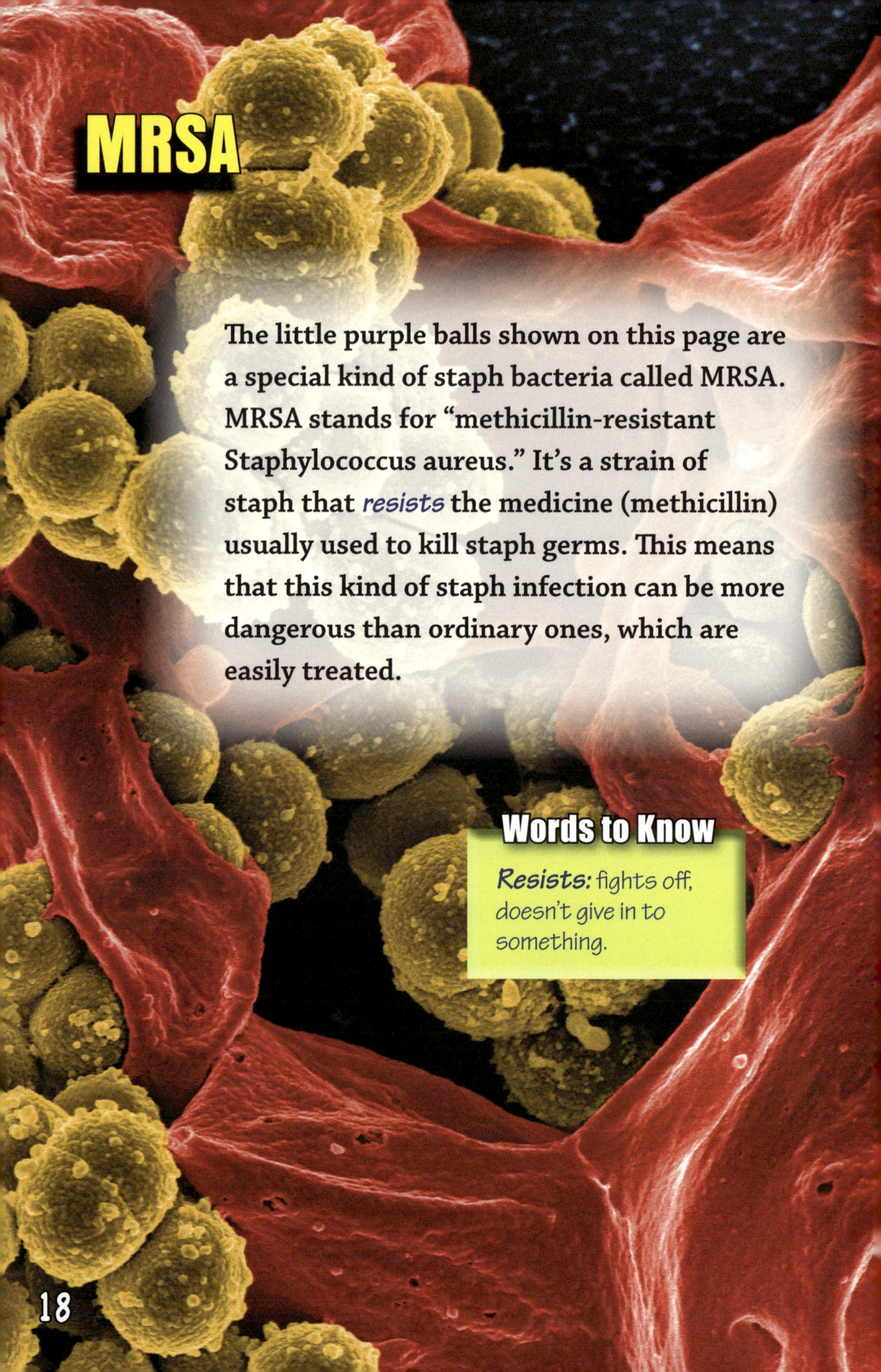

MRSA

The little purple balls shown on this page are a special kind of staph bacteria called MRSA. MRSA stands for "methicillin-resistant Staphylococcus aureus." It's a strain of staph that *resists* the medicine (methicillin) usually used to kill staph germs. This means that this kind of staph infection can be more dangerous than ordinary ones, which are easily treated.

Words to Know

Resists: fights off, doesn't give in to something.

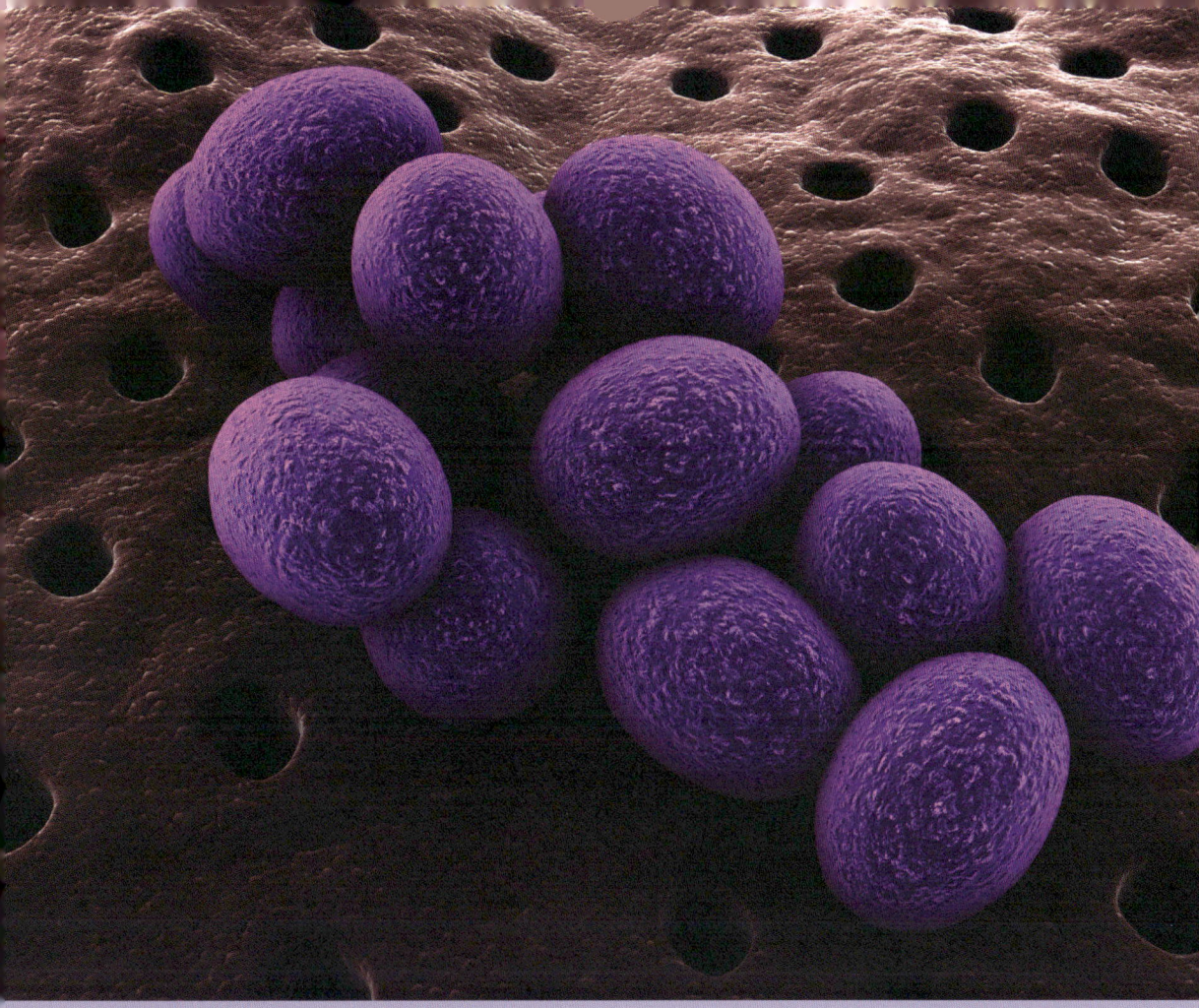

Like many other staph infections, MRSA generally starts as small red bumps that look like pimples or insect bites. These can quickly turn into deep, painful sores, like the one shown on this page. Sometimes the infection stays in the skin. If it's not treated, though, it can also move inside the body. Then it can cause infections in bones, joints, the bloodstream, and even your heart and lungs.

See a doctor if you have a sore that's red and warm, is oozing pus (a yellowish, white fluid), or if you have a fever. Although the medicines used to treat other staph infections won't work on MRSA, doctors do have other medicines that kill the MRSA bacteria.

Strep Infections

ASK THE DOCTOR

My mom thinks I have strep throat. How can I know for sure?

Answer: If you have a strep throat infection, you will have a red, painful throat. You may have white patches on your tonsils or swollen lymph nodes in your neck. You might run a fever and have a headache. The only way to know for sure that you have strep throat, though, is to go to your doctor. She will swab the back of your throat and do a test that tells her whether strep bacteria are present. If they are, she will have you take medicine that will kill the strep bacteria.

Like staph bacteria, streptococcus bacteria (shown above, usually called "strep" for short) can cause skin infections, sore throats, and upset stomachs. It can also cause more serious illnesses like *pneumonia.* Sore throats are the most common sickness strep causes.

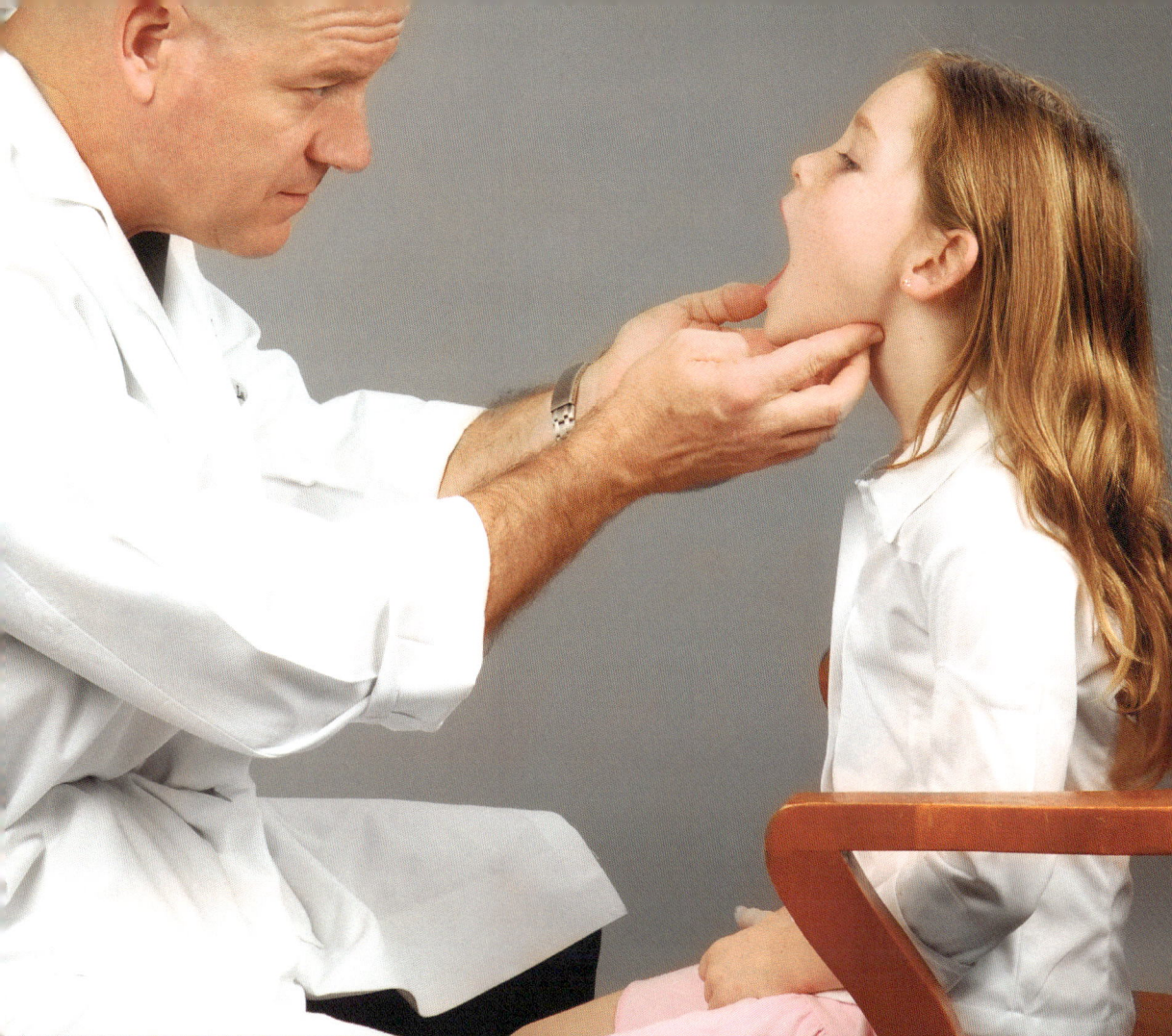

Words to Know

Pneumonia: a serious lung infection.

Inflammation: pain, swelling, redness, and heat in body tissues when they've been hurt.

Immune: protection against diseases.

A sore throat, also called a throat infection, is a painful *inflammation* of the throat, including the back of the tongue, the roof of the mouth, and the tonsils (the fleshy tissue that's part of the throat's *immune* defenses). Strep bacteria is just one of the germs that cause sore throats.

Stomach Upsets

Did You Know?

Some kinds of E. coli are actually good for you. In fact, we need E. coli and other kinds of bacteria in our intestines to help our bodies grow properly and stay healthy. Only certain kinds of E. coli produce toxins that make you sick.

Bacteria is often a common cause of stomach illnesses. For example, E. coli (shown above, short for Escherichia coli) is a bacteria that causes stomach cramps and diarrhea when it gets into your stomach and *intestines*. This infection is more common during the summer months. Over-the-counter medicines (like that shown on the next page) can help you feel better. Sometimes, though, you may also need to see a doctor.

The most common way to get E. coli is from food. It can also be easily spread from an infected person. To protect yourself from E. coli getting in your stomach and intestines (shown at right):

- Wash your hands carefully with soap before eating or handling food.
- Don't eat undercooked meat.
- Keep raw meat separate from other foods. Use hot water and soap to wash cutting boards and dishes if raw meat has touched them.
- Don't drink un*pasteurized* milk.
- Keep hot food hot and cold food cold. Refrigerate leftovers right away or throw them away.

Words to Know

Intestines: the tubes inside your belly that connect your stomach to the hole where your bowel movements leave your body.

Pasteurized: heated milk to kill bacteria.

Tuberculosis

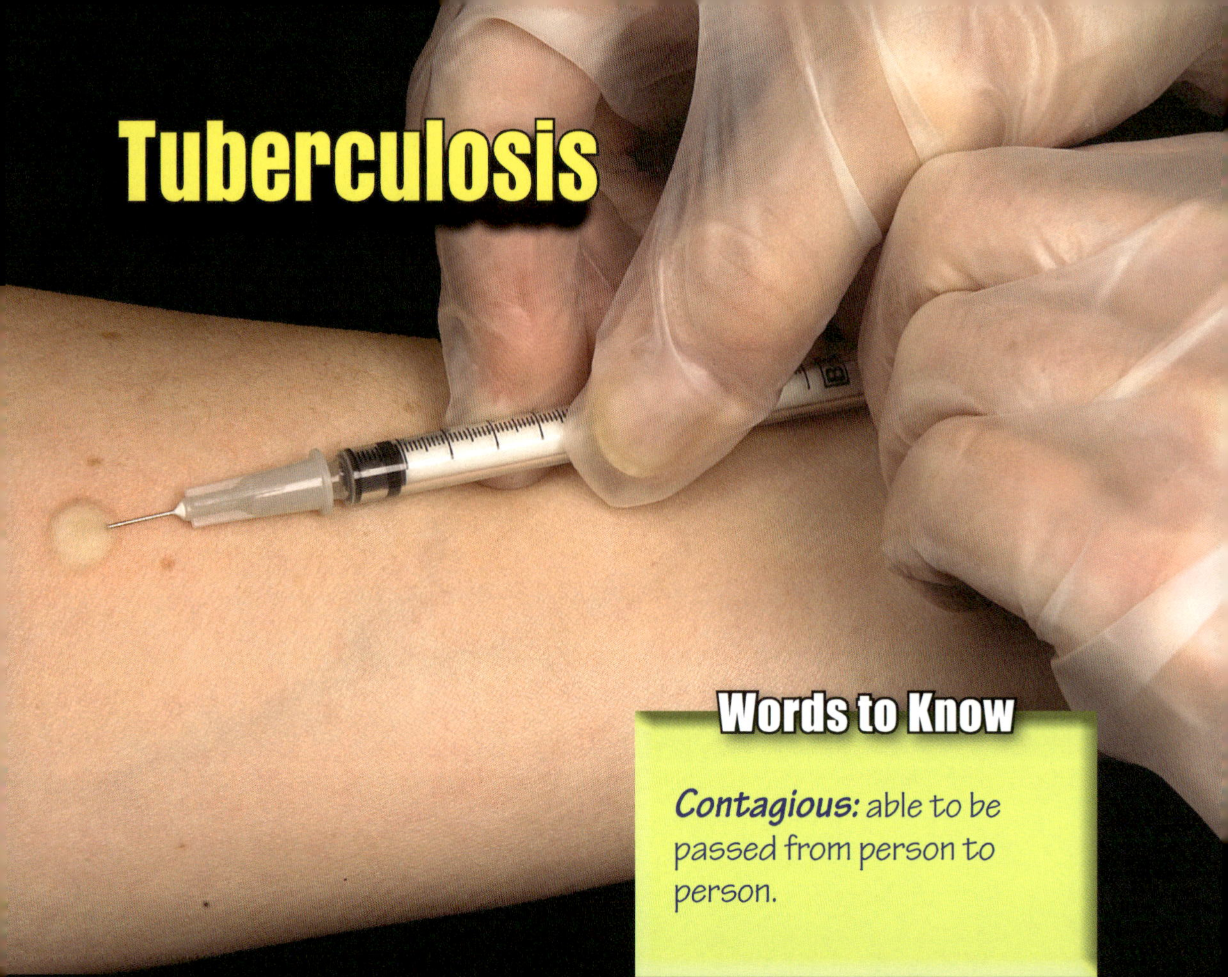

Words to Know

Contagious: able to be passed from person to person.

Tuberculosis (TB) is a *contagious* lung disease caused by bacteria (shown at right) that spread through the air. If people with TB bacteria in their lungs cough, sneeze, talk, or spit, they send the bacteria into the air.

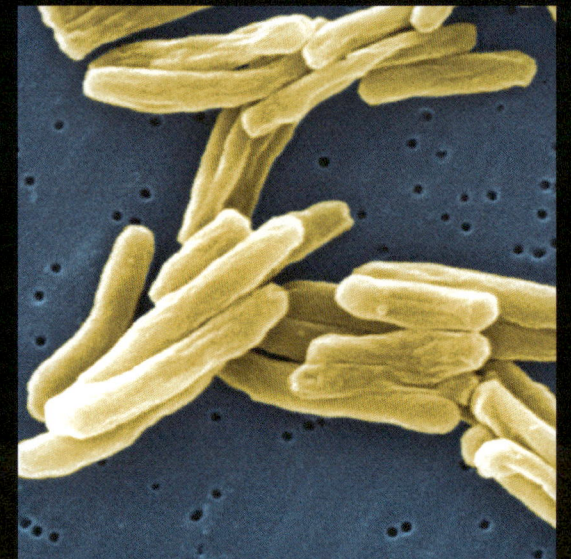

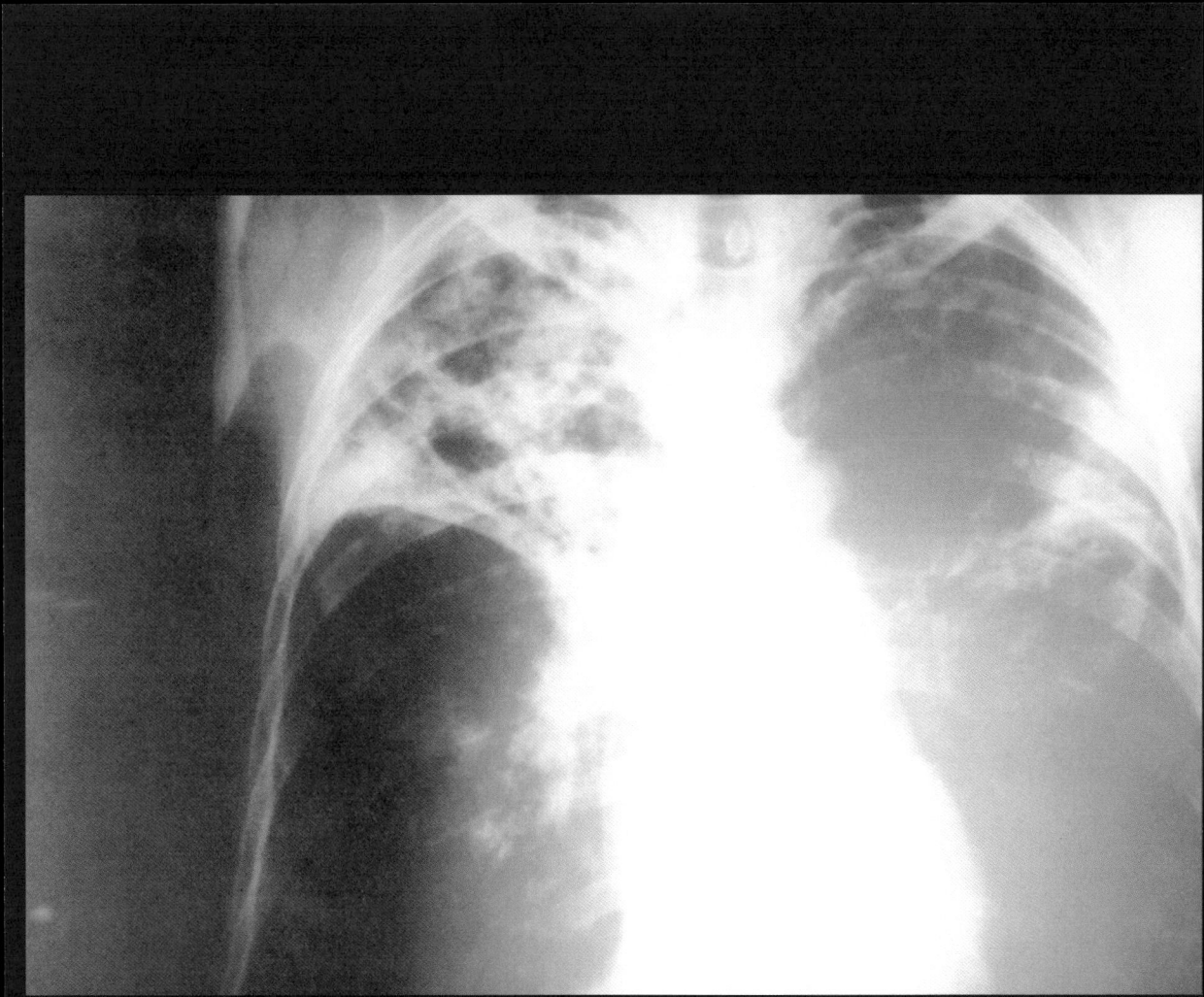

Anthrax

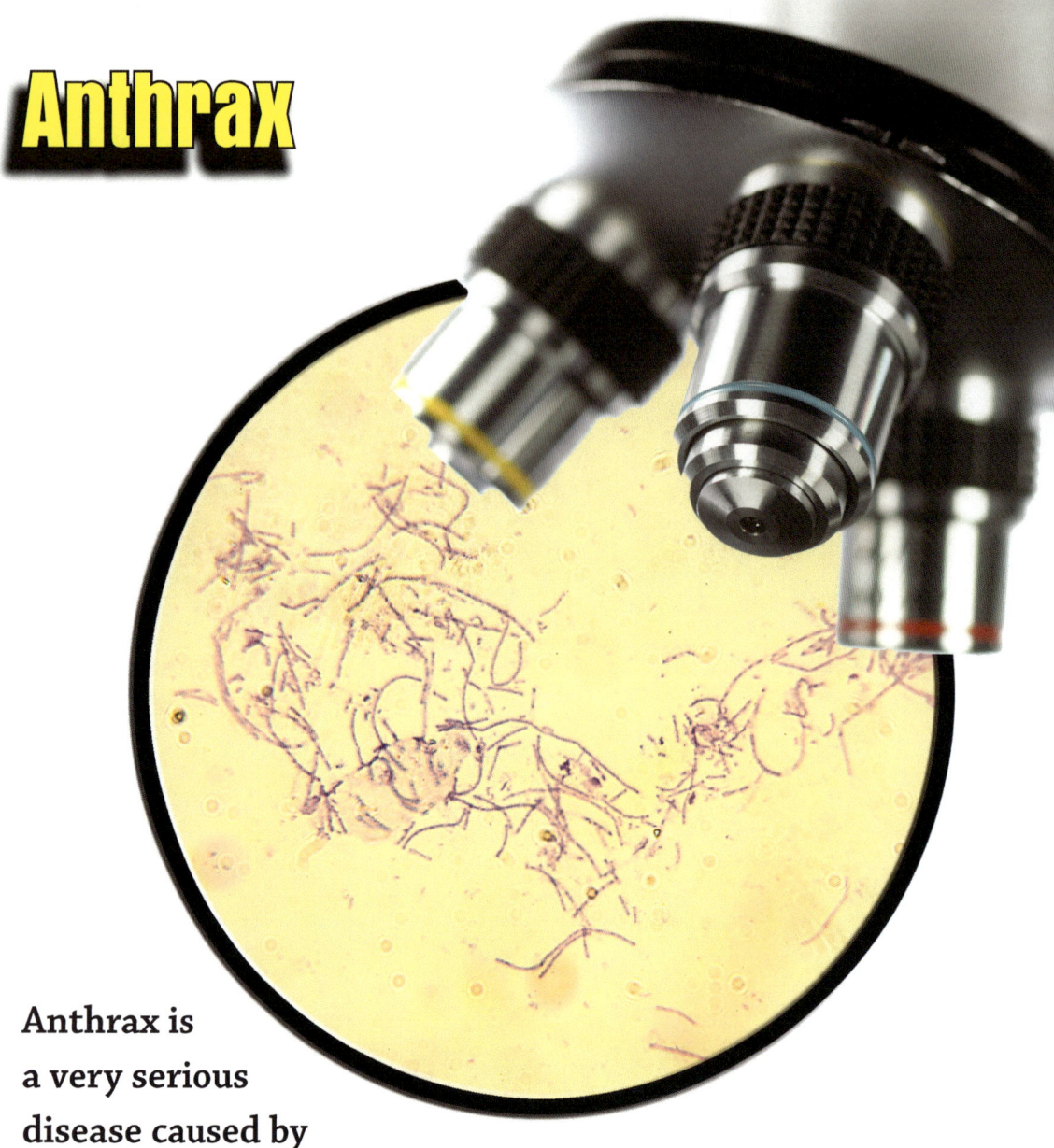

Anthrax is a very serious disease caused by the bacteria shown to the right. It can infect skin, lungs, stomach, and intestines.

People catch anthrax from animals—either by handling animal products like wool or eating undercooked meat from an animal that has the bacteria. If you think you've been *exposed* to anthrax, see your doctor. There are medicines that can cure this disease.

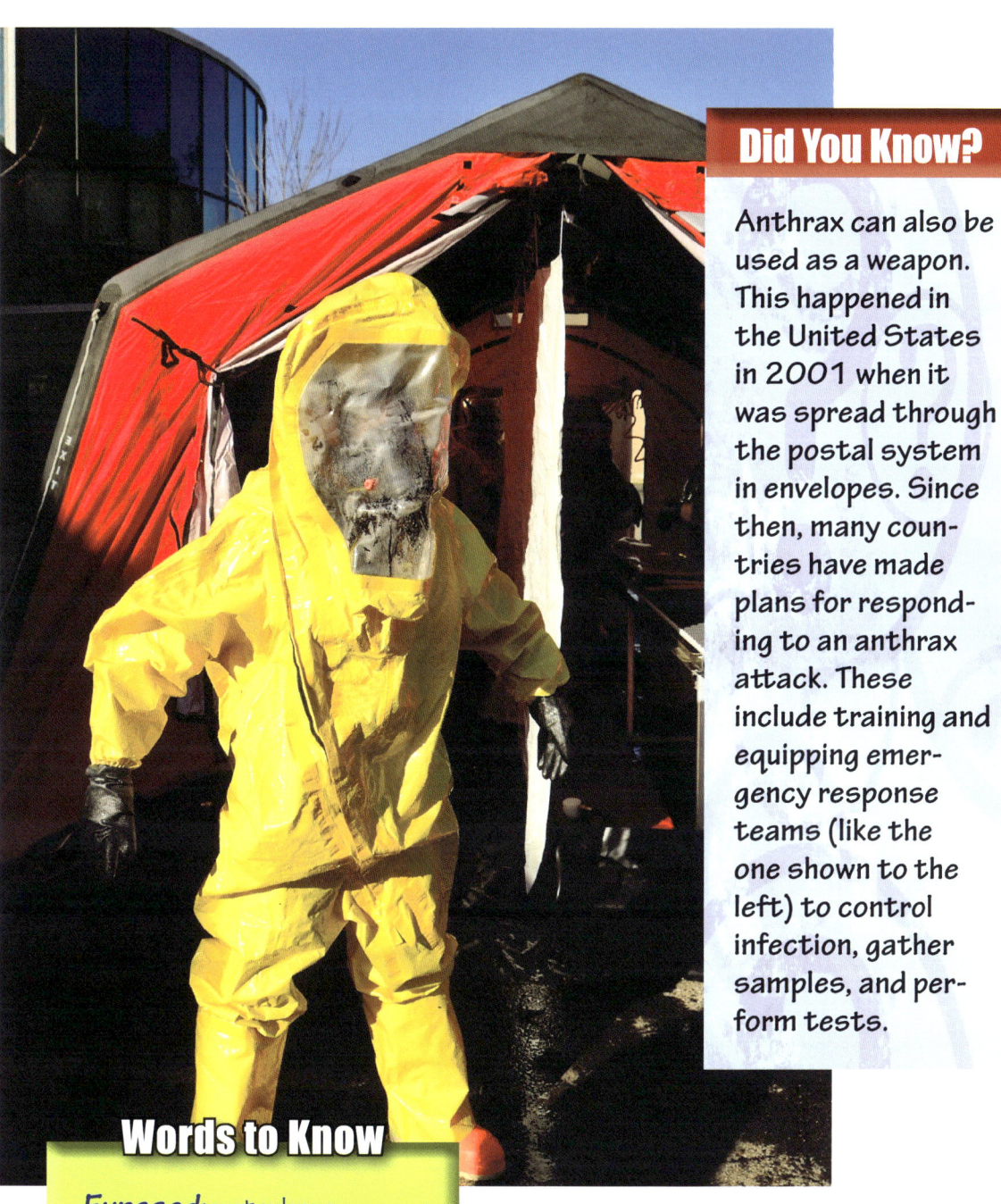

Did You Know?

Anthrax can also be used as a weapon. This happened in the United States in 2001 when it was spread through the postal system in envelopes. Since then, many countries have made plans for responding to an anthrax attack. These include training and equipping emergency response teams (like the one shown to the left) to control infection, gather samples, and perform tests.

Words to Know

Exposed: put where some action or influence can take place.

Treating Bacterial Infections

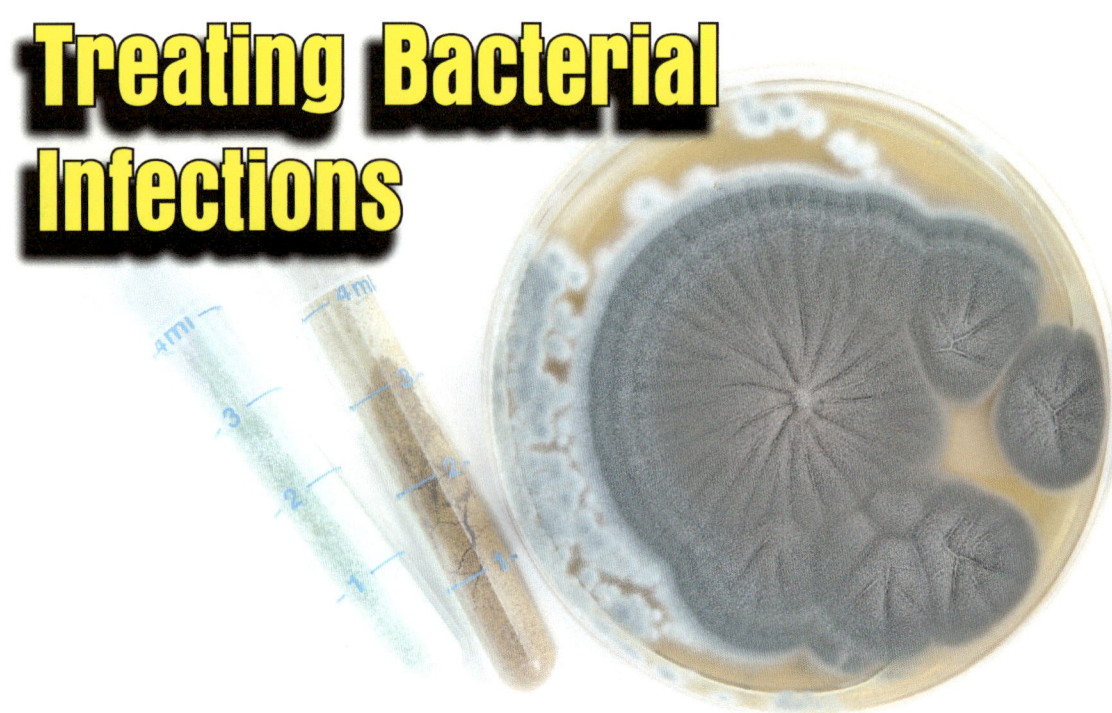

Once upon a time, many people died from bacterial infections that today we don't consider very serious at all. Then in the late 1800s, scientists accidentally discovered that a substance found in bread mold could kill certain bacteria. In 1942, doctors began to use the first antibiotic—penicillin. Today, antibiotics are among the medicines doctors use most often.

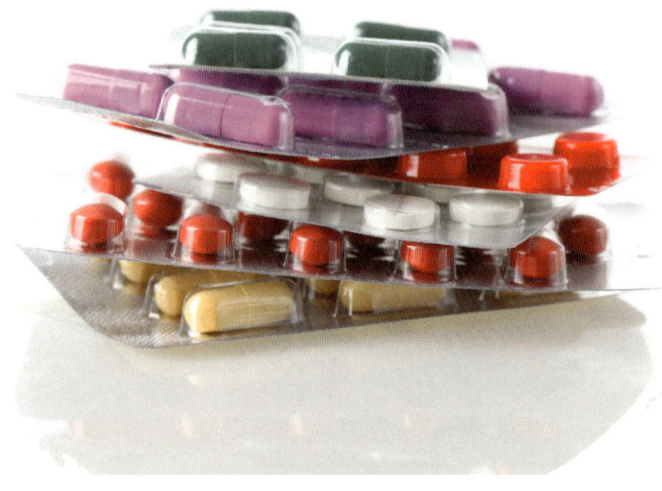

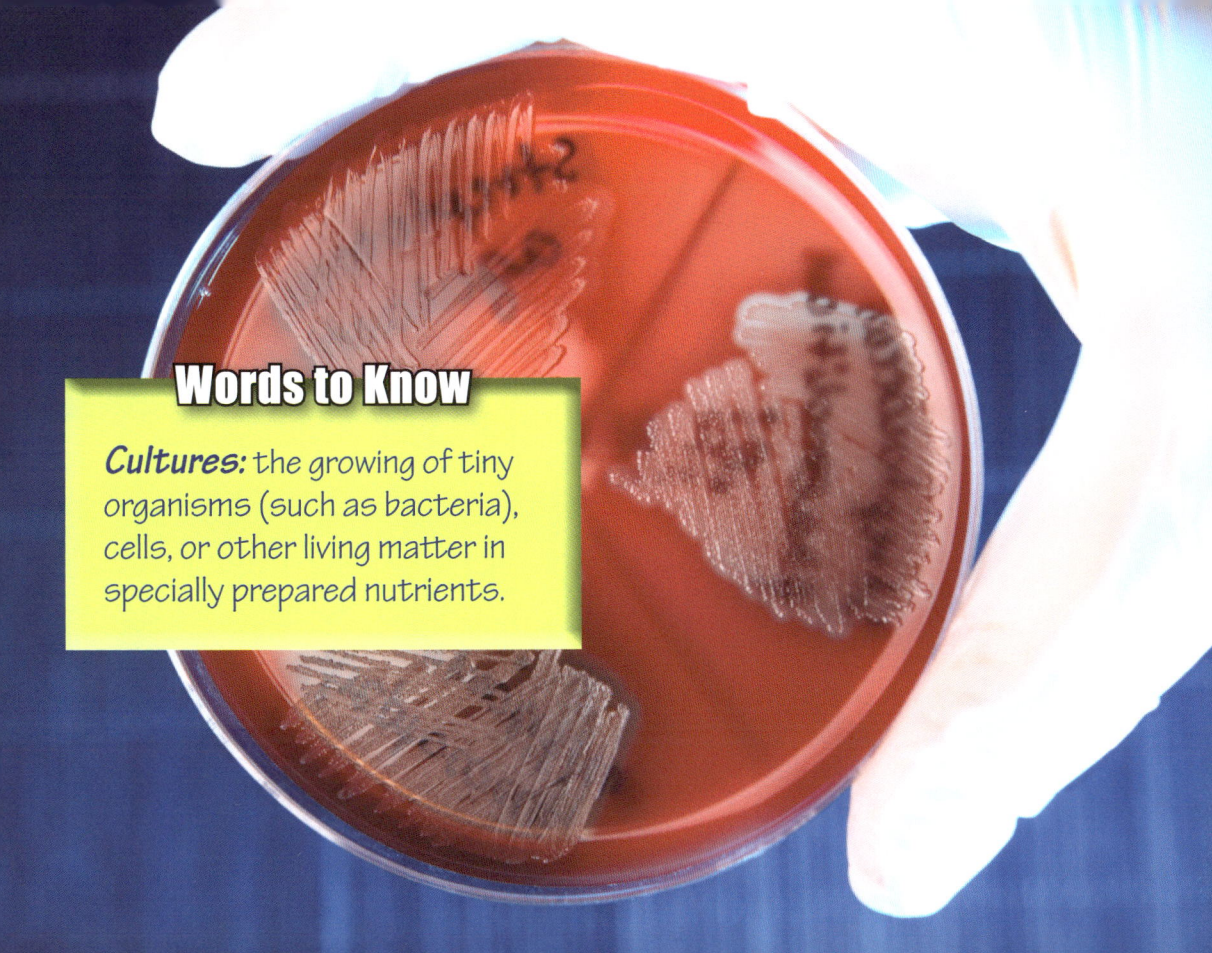

Words to Know

Cultures: the growing of tiny organisms (such as bacteria), cells, or other living matter in specially prepared nutrients.

More than 100 different antibiotics are available now. These medicines cure life-threatening infections—and small ones that may make you merely uncomfortable. They do so by killing or injuring bacteria. Not every antibiotic works with all bacteria, though. Doctors sometimes use bacteria *cultures* like the one shown in the dish above to see if a certain antibiotic will work against a particular bacteria.

People have become so used to taking antibiotics that they sometimes think there's a pill to cure every illness—but antibiotics only kill bacteria, not other kinds of germs.

The Problem with Antibiotics

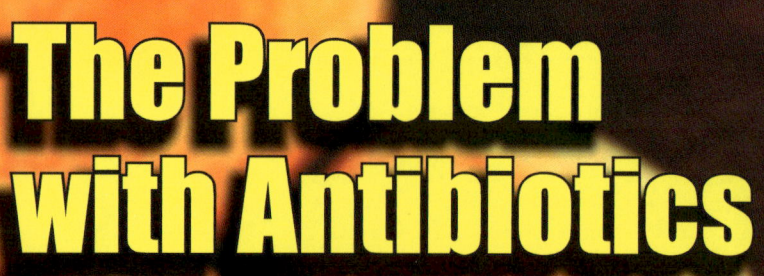

People have used antibiotics so much in the past sixty or so years that there's a problem: Bacteria have begun to change. Some of them can now resist antibiotics. MRSA, which we talked about earlier, is an example of a bacteria that no longer responds to some antibiotic medicines.

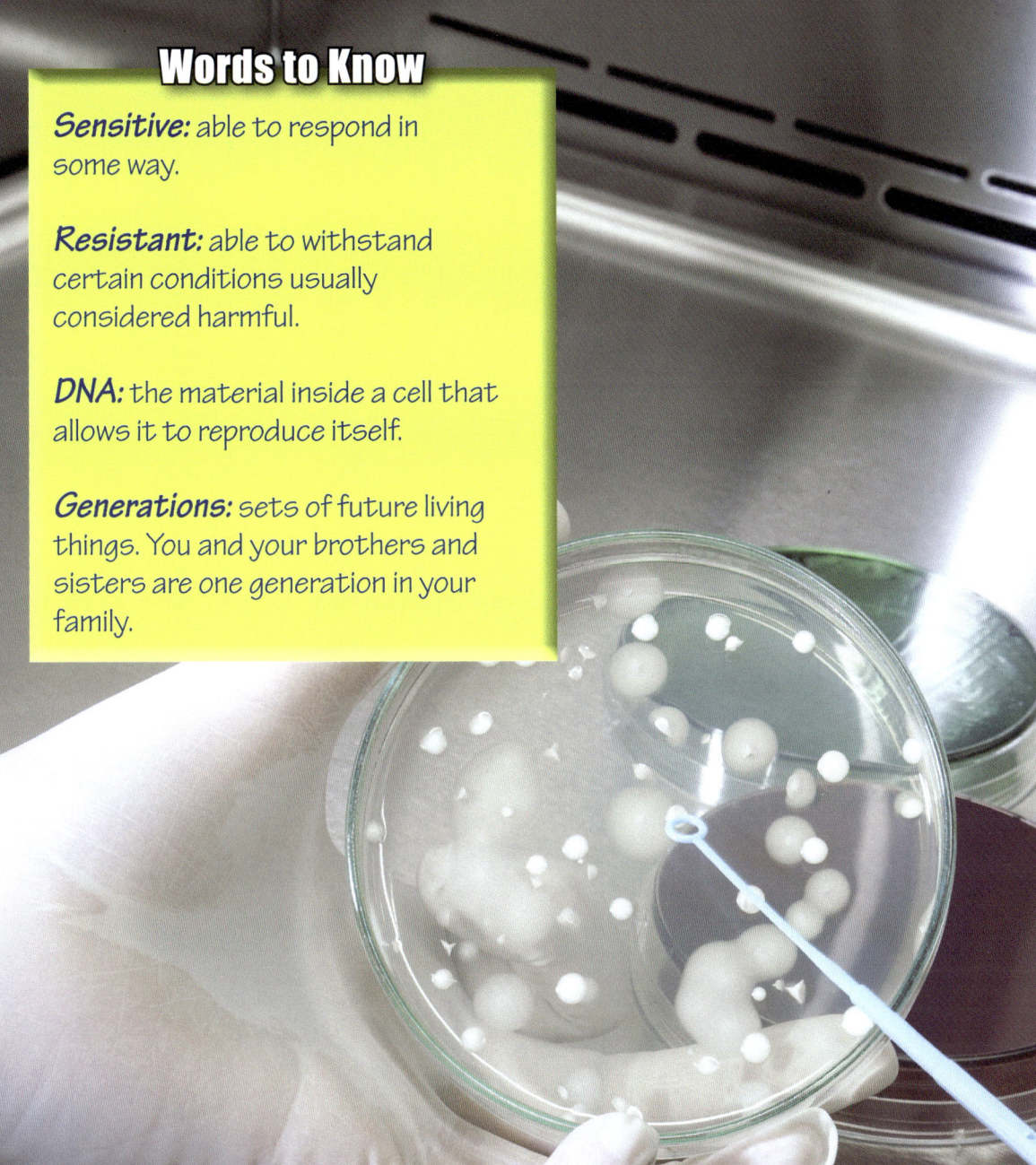

Words to Know

Sensitive: able to respond in some way.

Resistant: able to withstand certain conditions usually considered harmful.

DNA: the material inside a cell that allows it to reproduce itself.

Generations: sets of future living things. You and your brothers and sisters are one generation in your family.

Every time a person takes antibiotics, *sensitive* bacteria are killed. Meanwhile, *resistant* germs may be left to grow. Using antibiotics too often increases these drug-resistant bacteria. This happens because the "weak" bacteria are killed, leaving the "strong" bacteria to pass along their *DNA* to future *generations* of bacteria (as illustrated on this page).

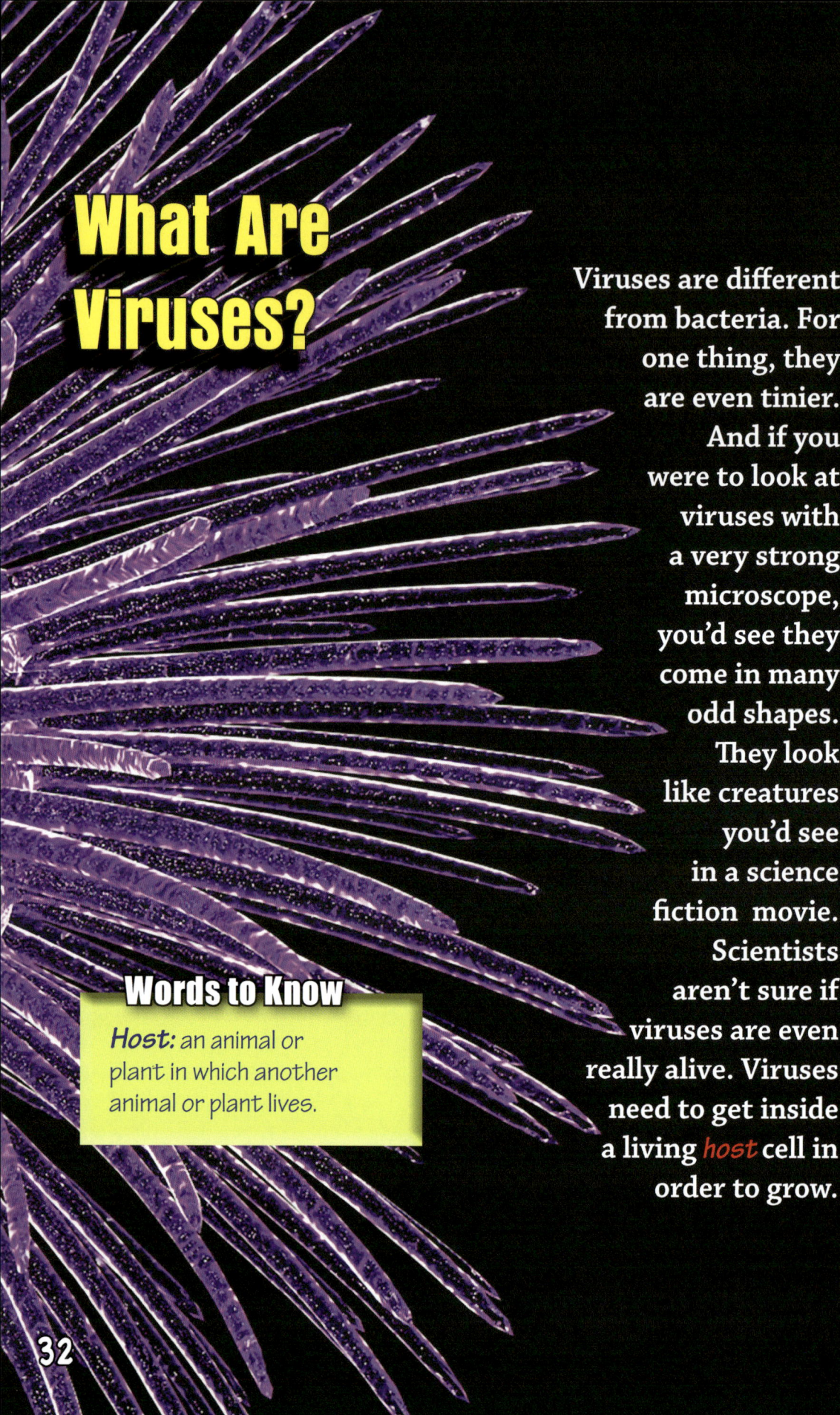

What Are Viruses?

Viruses are different from bacteria. For one thing, they are even tinier. And if you were to look at viruses with a very strong microscope, you'd see they come in many odd shapes. They look like creatures you'd see in a science fiction movie. Scientists aren't sure if viruses are even really alive. Viruses need to get inside a living *host* cell in order to grow.

Words to Know

Host: an animal or plant in which another animal or plant lives.

Here are some of viruses' strange shapes.

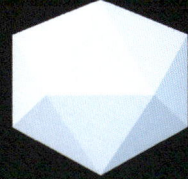

Papillomavirus
Enterovirus
Rhinovirus
Rotavirus

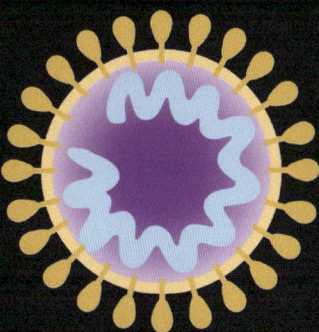

Coronavirus

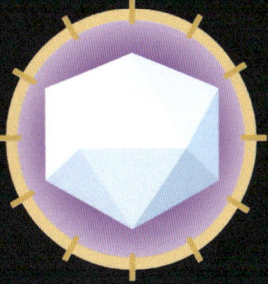

Herpesvirus
Hepatitis B virus

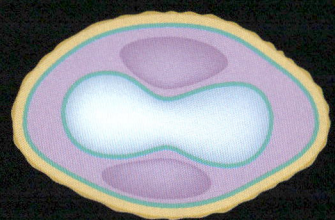

Smallpox virus

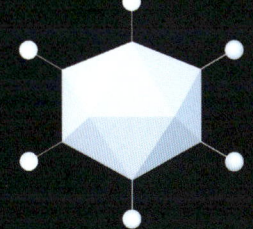

Mastadenovirus

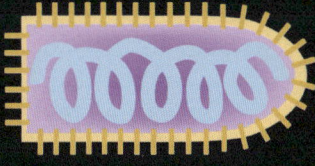

Rabies virus

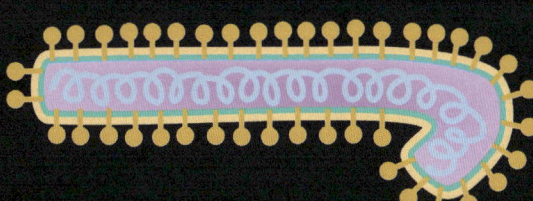

Filovirus (Ebola virus)

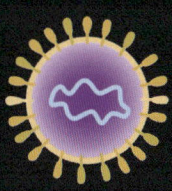

Hepatitis D virus

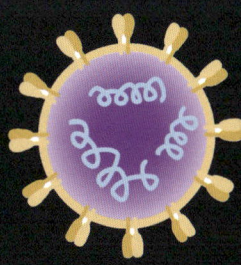

Hantavirus

33

How Do Viruses Make You Sick?

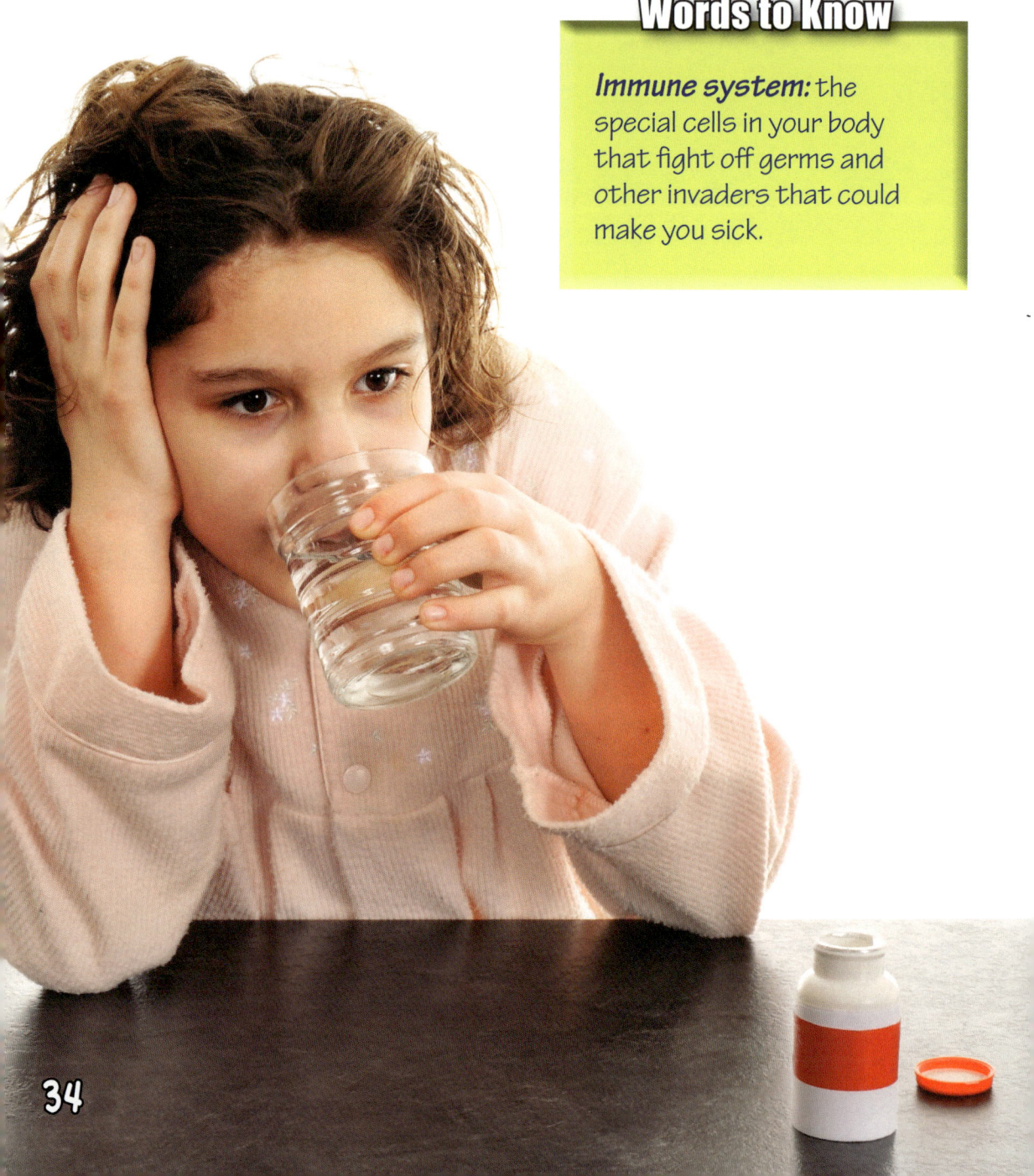

Words to Know

Immune system: the special cells in your body that fight off germs and other invaders that could make you sick.

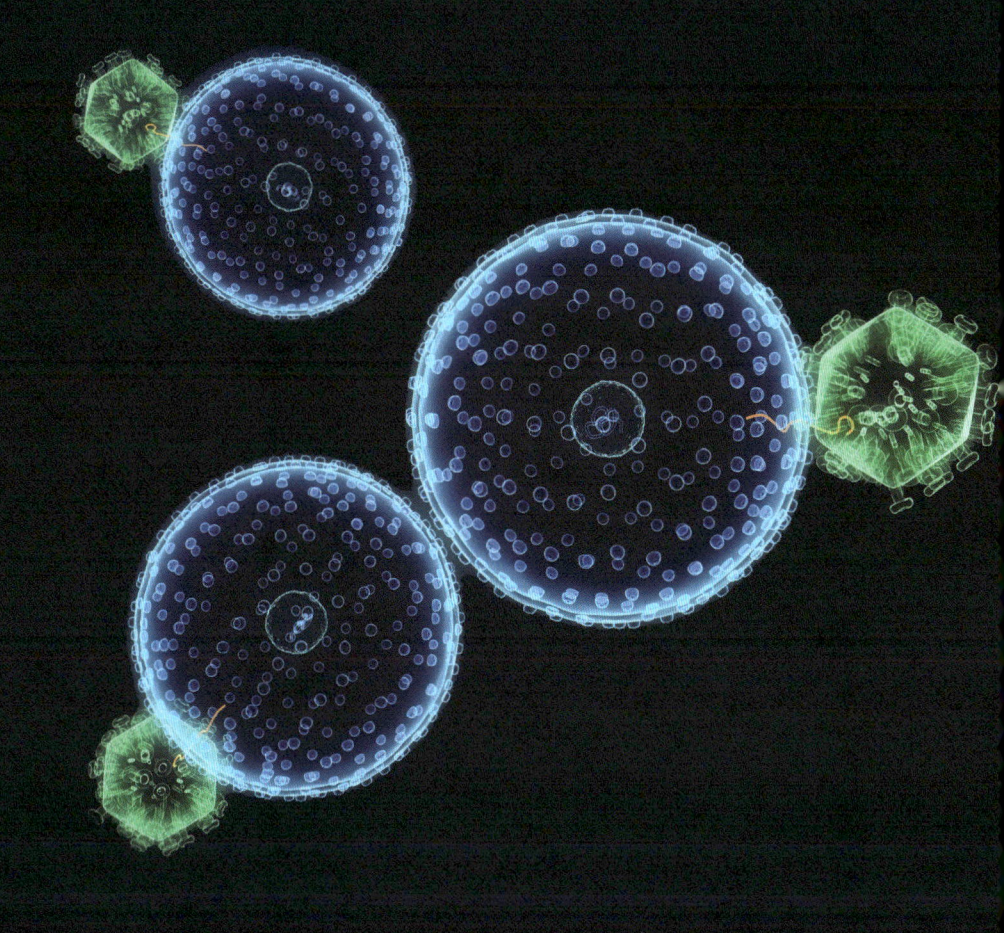

When a virus takes over a cell, it kills it or upsets the way it works. The green cells shown here are viruses sticking themselves into normal, healthy cells. When this happens, you get sick. Because the viruses are inside your cells, your *immune system* has to kill those cells in order to kill the viruses. When your cells die, you may feel sick. Your body may also get a fever because viruses don't grow as well at higher temperatures.

The Common Cold

The common cold is an illness caused by a viral infection in the nose. These viruses can also get into the *sinuses*, ears, and the tubes in your lungs. The *symptoms* of a cold include sneezing, runny nose, stuffy nose, sore or scratchy throat, and cough. Sometimes, a cold may also give you a headache, fever, and body aches.

Colds last on average for one week. Mild colds may last only two or three days. Bad colds can last up to two weeks.

Did You Know?

On average, adults get two to three colds per year, while children get six to ten.

Your dog or cat can't catch your cold. Only human beings get colds.

More than a hundred different viruses cause colds. Rhinoviruses (shown on the right) are the most common. They cause at least one-half of all colds.

Like all viruses, cold viruses can only grow when they are inside living cells. When they're on a surface (like a doorknob or a telephone), they cannot grow. As soon as they get inside your nose, though, they come alive.

Cold symptoms are mostly caused by what your body does to fight the virus. Your nose makes more *mucus*. You sneeze and cough. All these things are your body's way of getting rid of the virus.

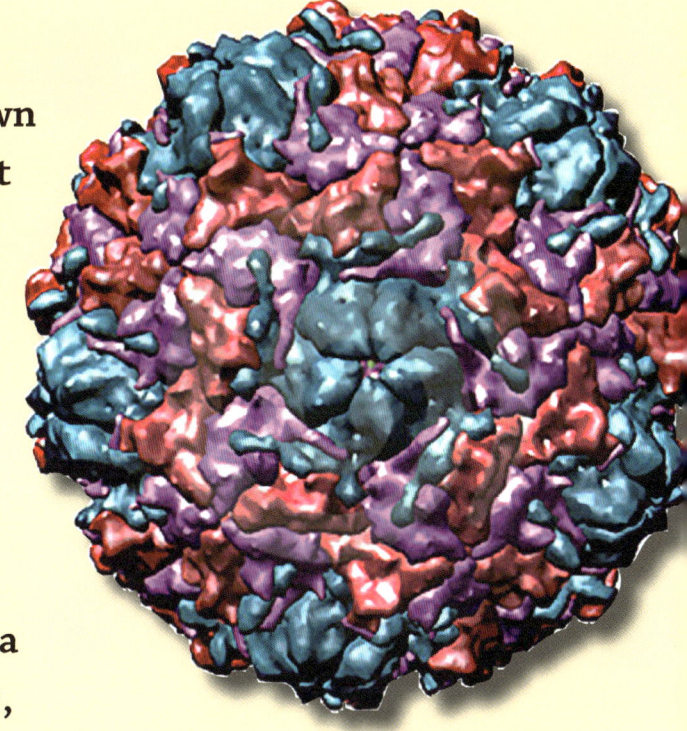

Words to Know

Sinuses: the holes inside the front of your skull.

Symptoms: the signs of an illness.

Mucus: a thick, slippery body fluid.

Pinkeye

ASK THE DOCTOR

If my little sister has pinkeye, will I get it?

Answer: You might! You get pinkeye by touching an infected person or something an infected person has touched, such as a used tissue. In the summertime, pinkeye can spread when kids share towels. It also can be spread through coughing and sneezing. The best way to keep from getting pinkeye is to wash your hands often with warm water and soap. Don't share your sister's washcloth, towel, drinking glass, or silverware.

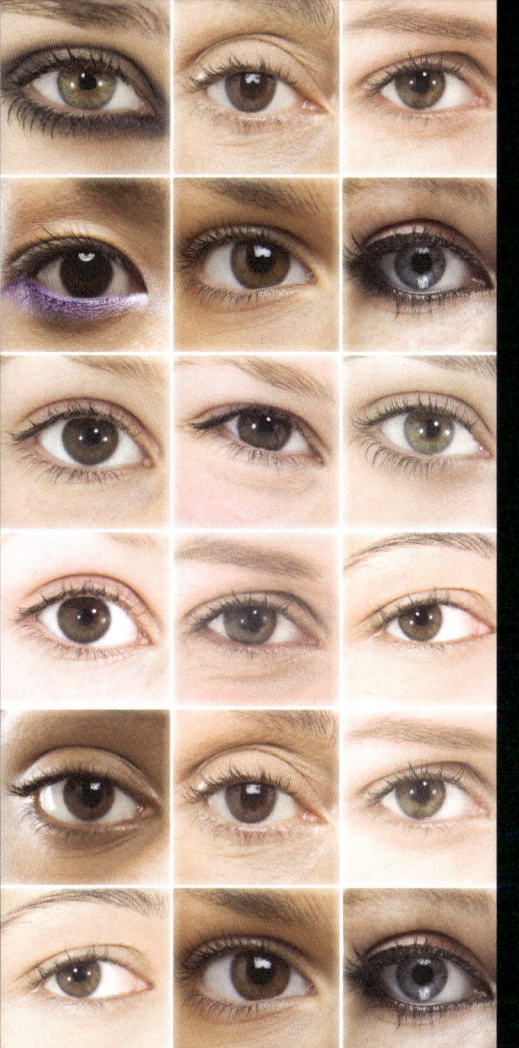

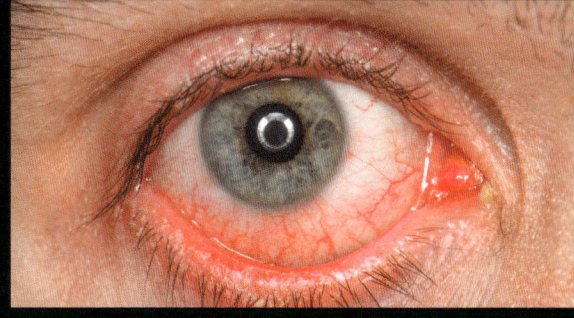

Healthy eyes, like those pictured to the left, come in many shapes and colors. Normally, the part of your eye around the *iris* is clear and white. But when the clear *membrane* that covers the white part becomes infected, the white part will look red (like the eye above), and it will feel sore and scratchy. This is called pinkeye. Your doctor may call it conjunctivitis. The same virus that causes the common cold can also cause pinkeye.

Words to Know

Iris: the colored part of your eye.

Membrane: a thin, flexible layer.

39

The Flu

Words to Know

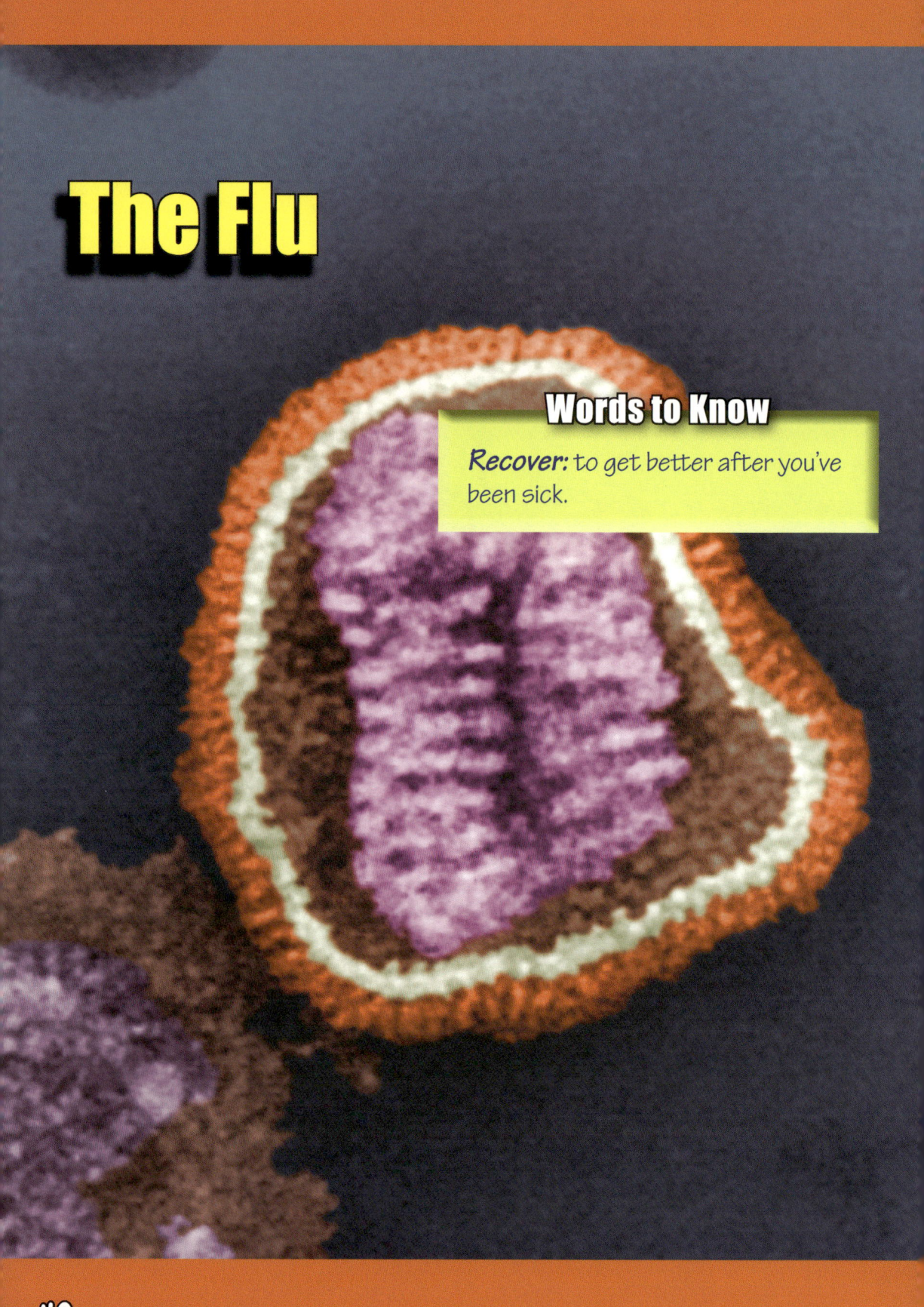

Recover: to get better after you've been sick.

Influenza ("flu" for short) is caused by the virus pictured to the left. It causes an illness that is much like the common cold. The flu is worse, though, and it usually lasts longer than a cold. People with the flu usually have a fever. Their bodies ache, and they may feel very tired.

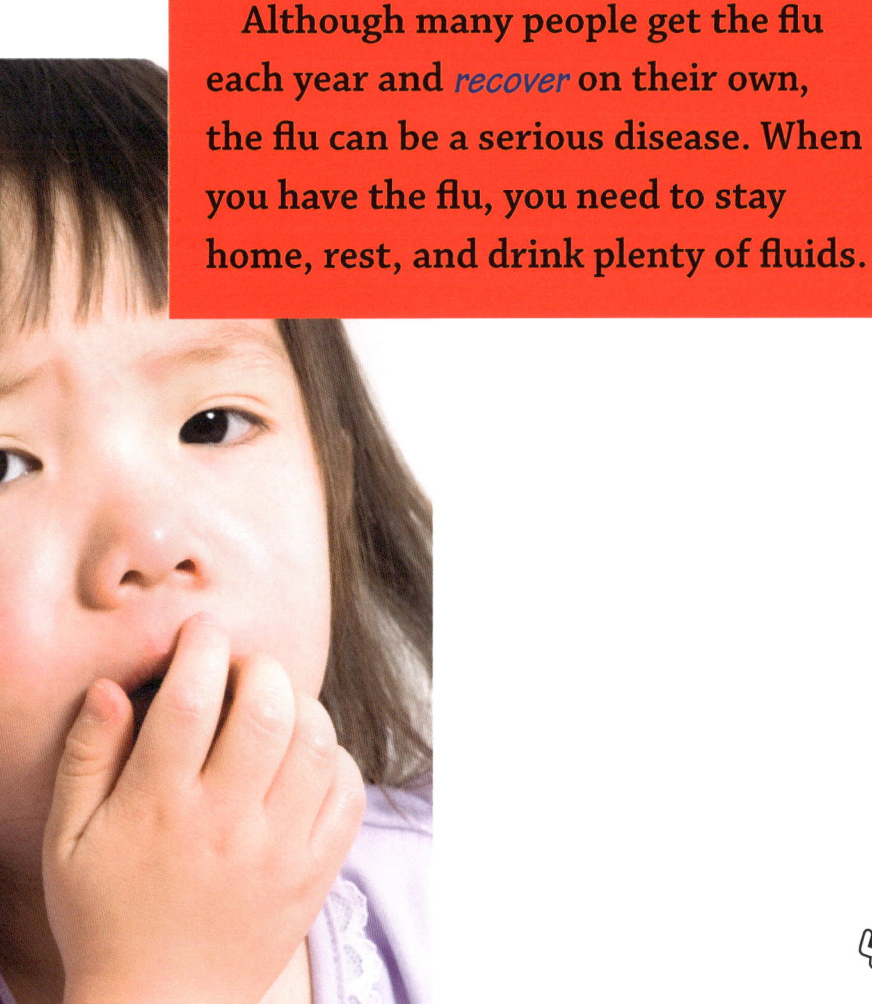

Although many people get the flu each year and *recover* on their own, the flu can be a serious disease. When you have the flu, you need to stay home, rest, and drink plenty of fluids.

Herpes

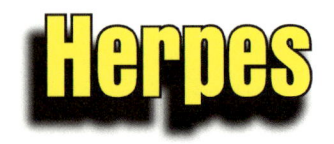

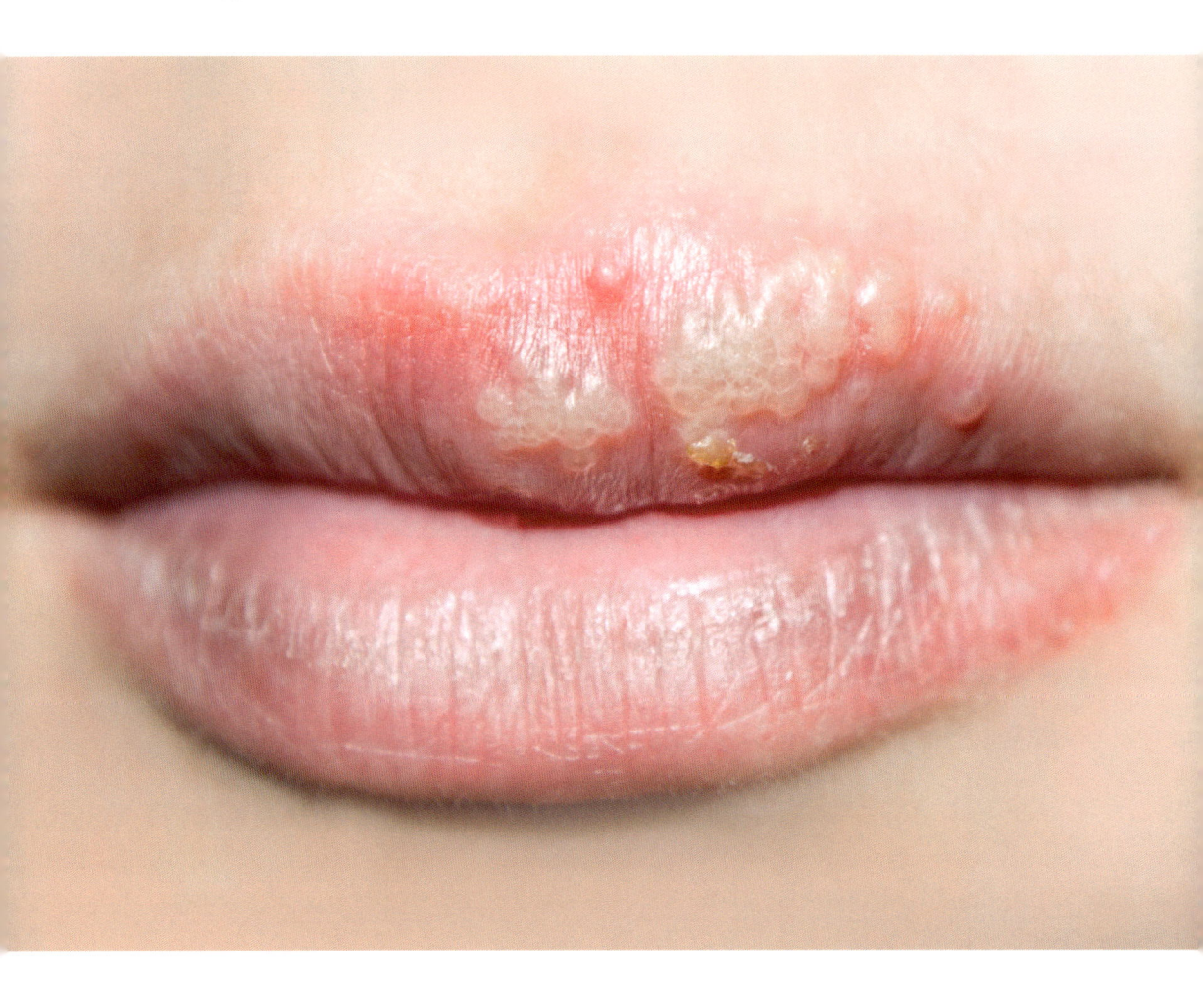

Herpes is another virus. There are several kinds of herpes viruses, but one of the most common is called *herpes simplex* (shown on the next page). It causes cold sores like the one shown above. Your body can't completely kill these viruses, so once you've had a cold sore, you're likely to get one again, often in the same spot. Protect yourself from catching herpes viruses by not sharing lipstick, utensils, or drinks with anyone who has a cold sore. And don't kiss them on the lips either!

Did You Know?

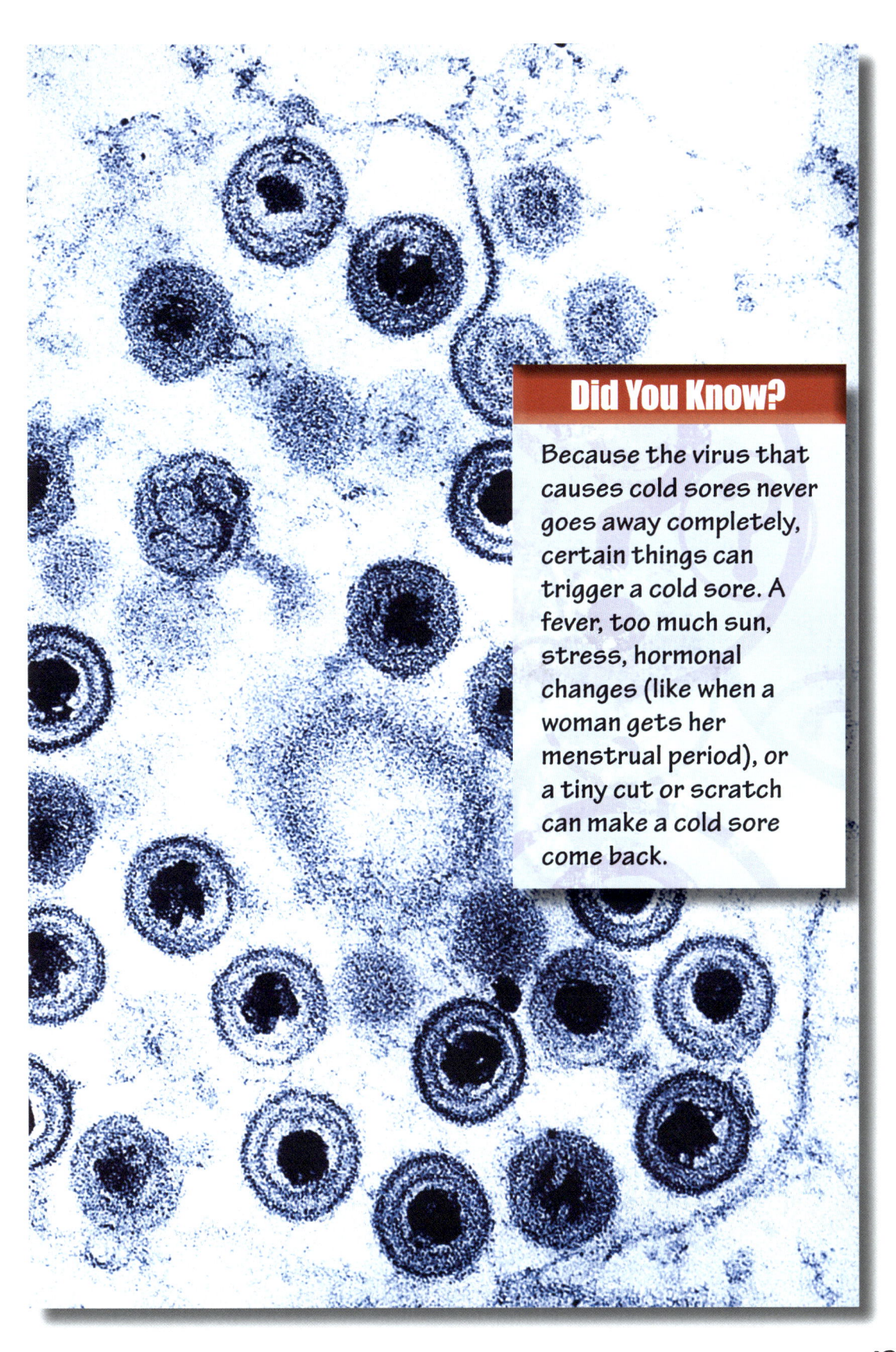

Because the virus that causes cold sores never goes away completely, certain things can trigger a cold sore. A fever, too much sun, stress, hormonal changes (like when a woman gets her menstrual period), or a tiny cut or scratch can make a cold sore come back.

West Nile Virus

West Nile virus (shown on the next page) has been found in humans, birds, horses, and other animals in Africa, Eastern Europe, the United States, and the Middle East. Mosquitoes get the virus inside them when they feed on birds that have it. The mosquitoes can then pass West Nile virus to humans and animals.

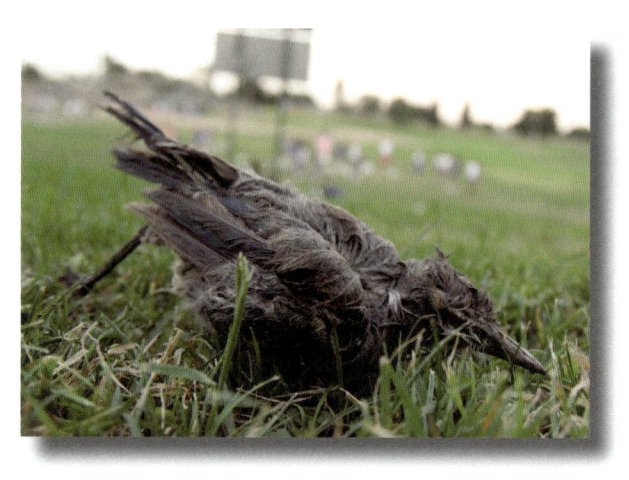

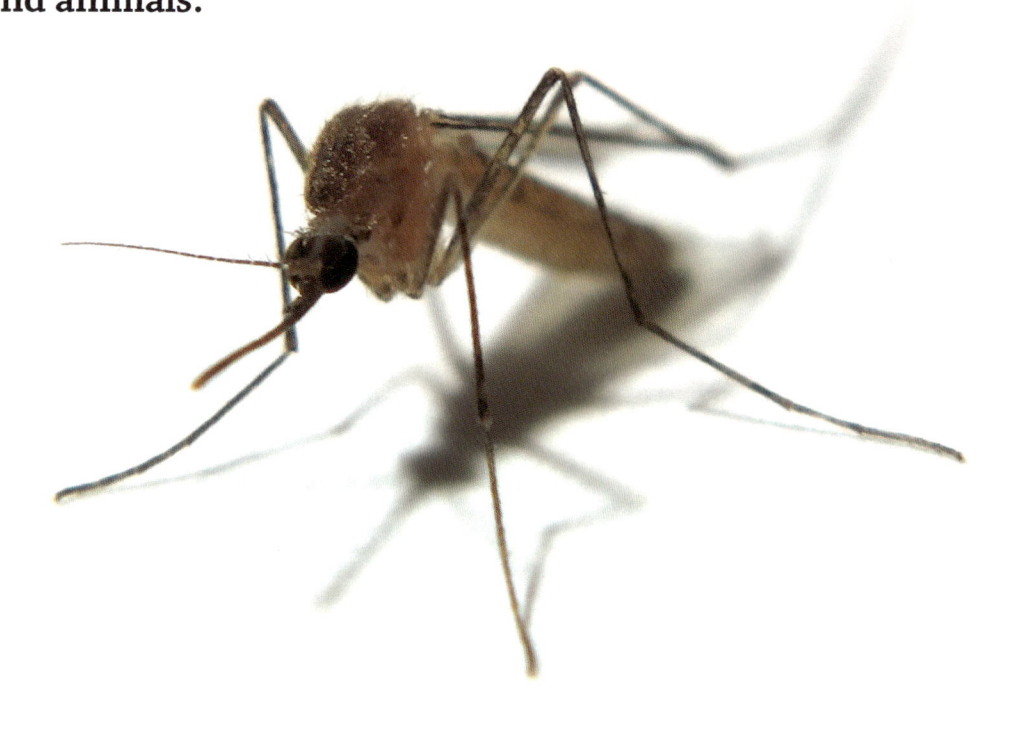

Did You Know?

Most people *infected* with West Nile virus will not have any signs of illness at all. People who do get sick often have only mild symptoms, such as fever, headache, and body aches. A few people who have the virus, however, may develop worse symptoms. People over fifty years of age are most at risk for having a serious sickness.

Words to Know

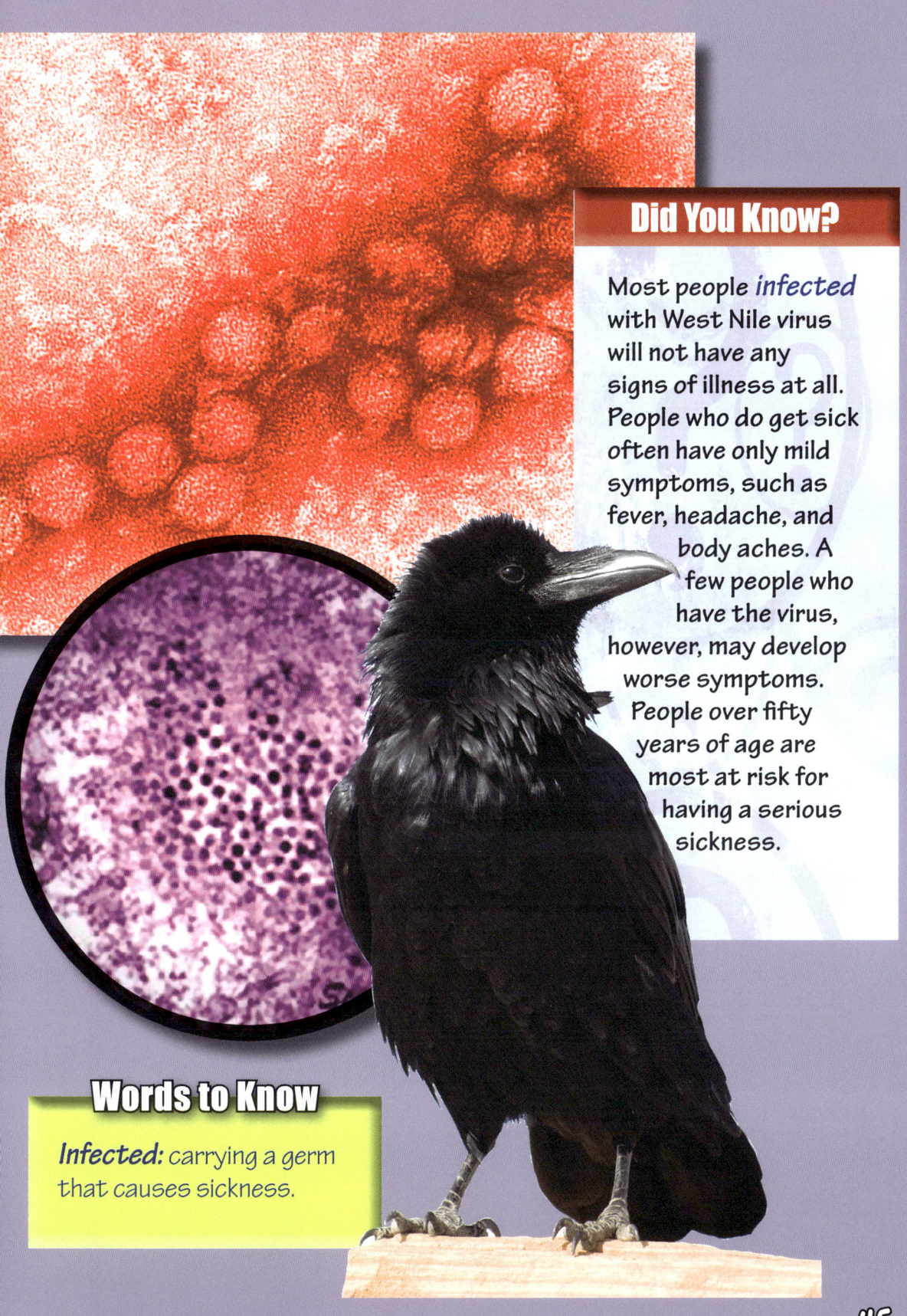

Infected: carrying a germ that causes sickness.

HIV

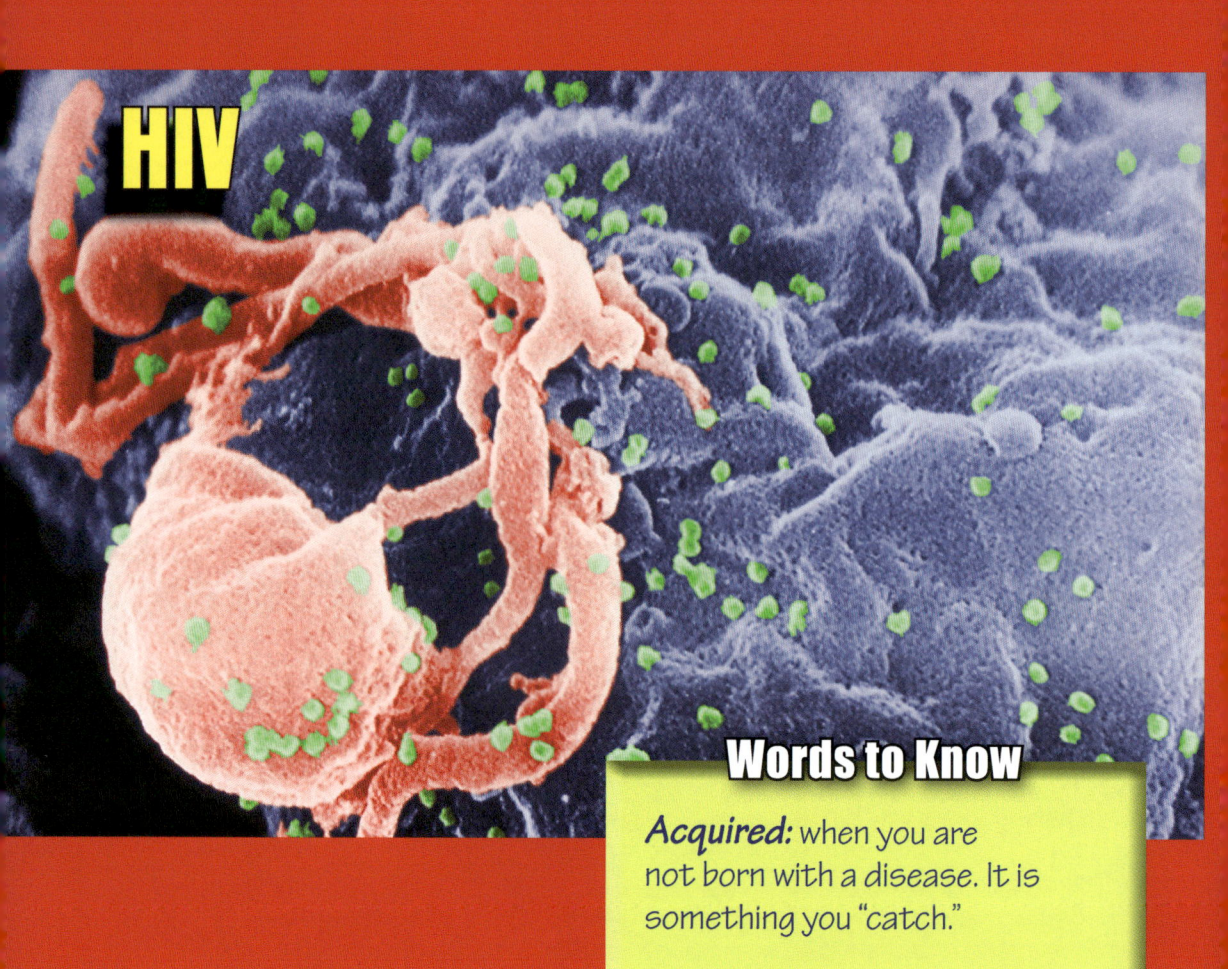

HIV (human immunodeficiency virus, shown above) causes AIDS (*acquired immunodeficiency syndrome*), a disease that damages white blood cells. These cells are an important part of the body's immune system. Scientists are working to find a cure for HIV, but so far they can only keep people who have it healthy longer.

Words to Know

Acquired: when you are not born with a disease. It is something you "catch."

Immunodeficiency: a lack in your immune system.

Syndrome: a set of symptoms that tend to occur together, although scientists do not understand exactly why.

Did You Know?

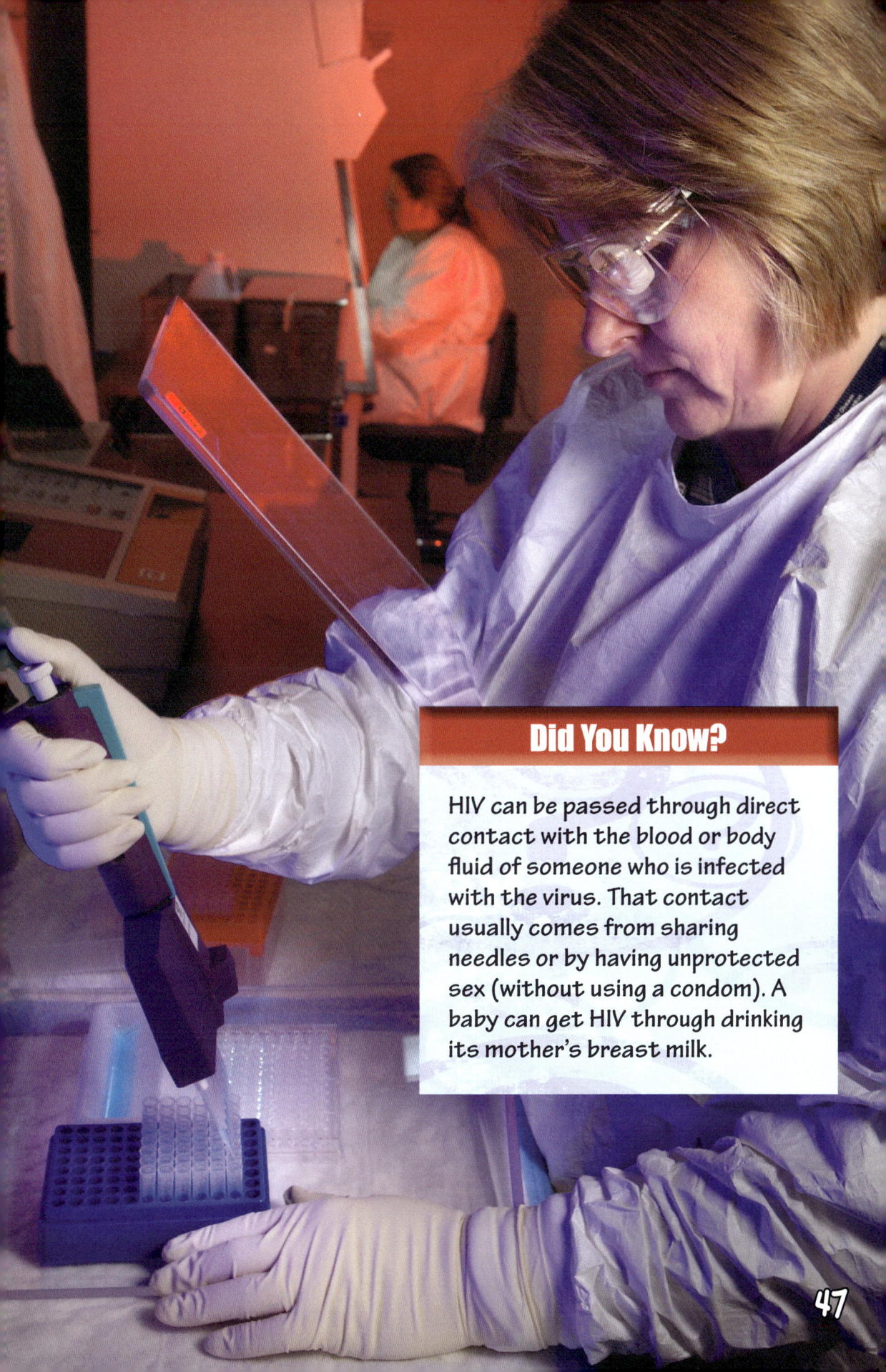

HIV can be passed through direct contact with the blood or body fluid of someone who is infected with the virus. That contact usually comes from sharing needles or by having unprotected sex (without using a condom). A baby can get HIV through drinking its mother's breast milk.

Treatment for Viral Diseases

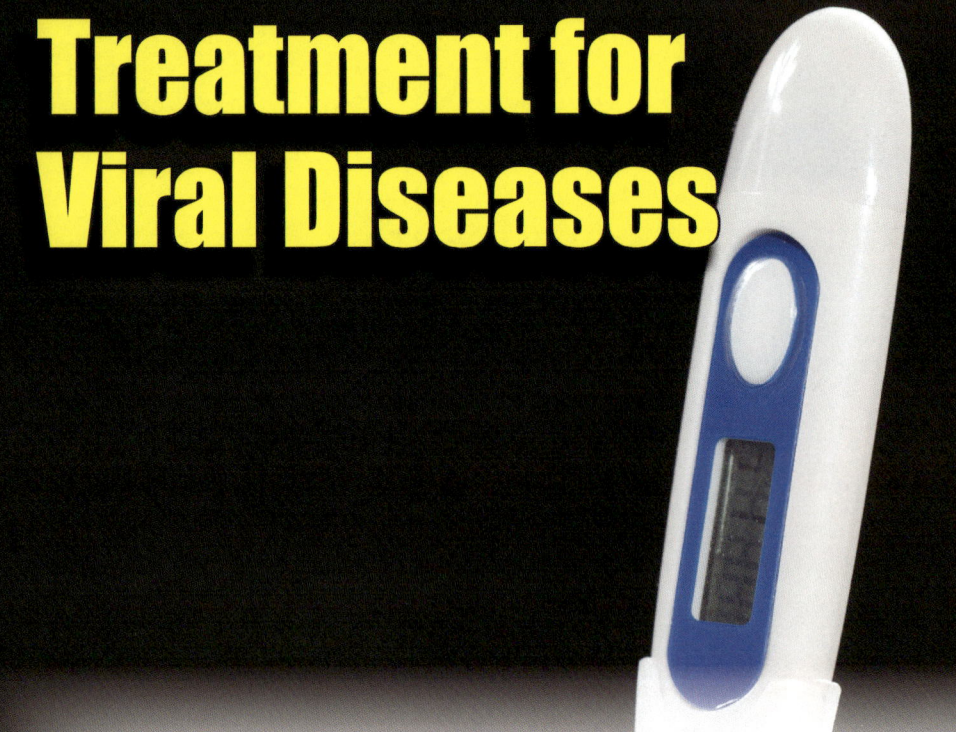

In most cases, there are no medicines that cure viruses. Your doctor may tell you to take a medicine like acetaminophen or ibuprofen that will ease aches and pains. Cough medications and decongestants can also help you cope with a viral infection like a cold or the flu. In the end, though, you usually just have to wait it out. You have to let your body fight off the virus.

In most cases, it's a job your body can handle all by itself. Some viruses are so serious or life-threatening, however (like HIV, for example), that scientists are working to find cures for them.

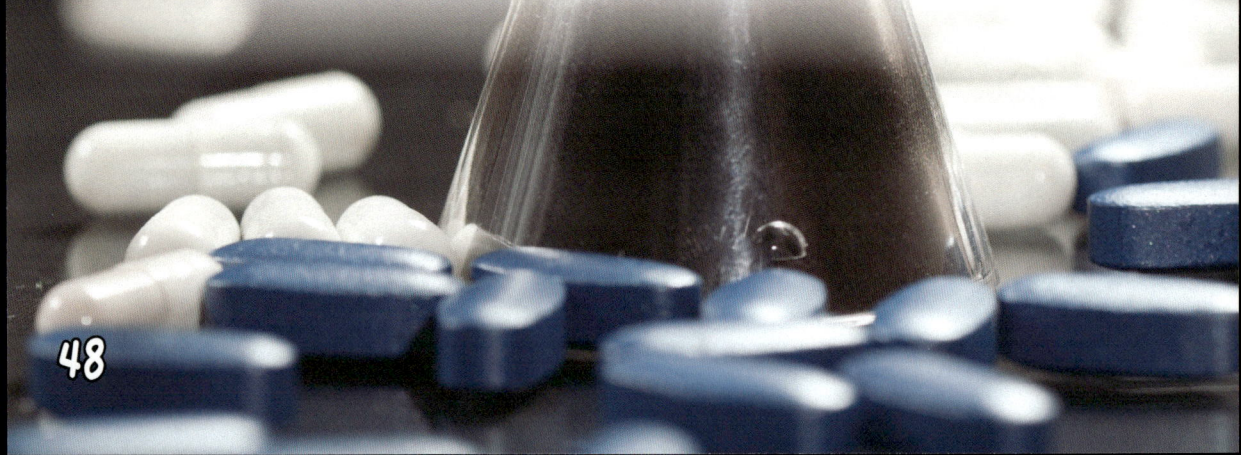

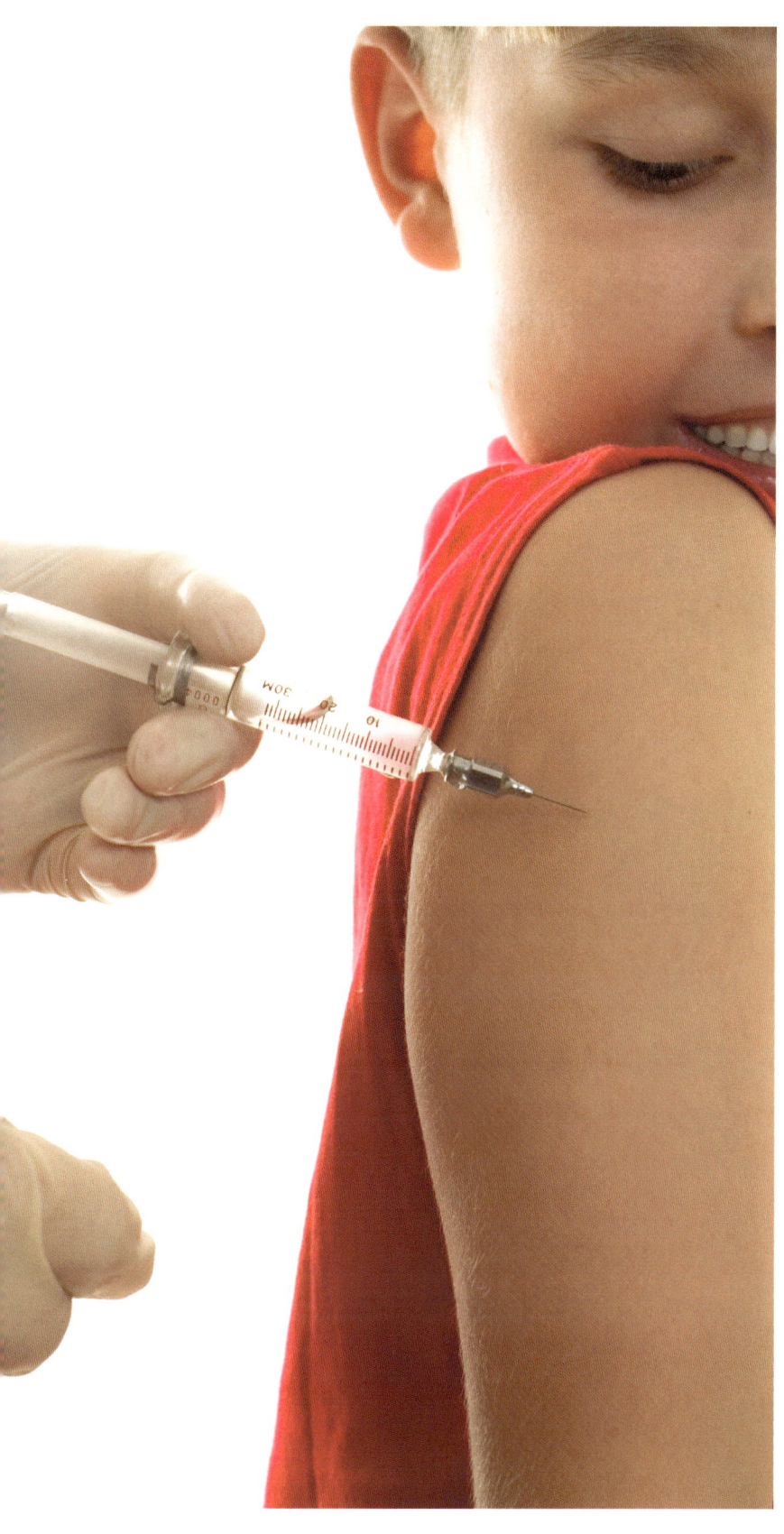

A few antiviral medicines have been developed that prevent viruses from growing more viruses. This makes the illness run its course more quickly. These remedies only work for a very few viruses. Vaccines have also been developed to protect people from getting viruses in the first place (like the flu vaccine, for instance, that's shown here).

Research

If you had lived two hundred years ago, the chances would have been high that you might have died from a viral or bacterial disease before you reached your fifth birthday. Scientists changed the world when they discovered new ways to fight diseases. These medicines give children the chance to grow up.

Today, scientists are still looking for new and better ways to fight germs. Recently, researchers developed a vaccine that will keep babies from getting ear infections. Meanwhile, scientists around the world are still working hard to find a cure for HIV.

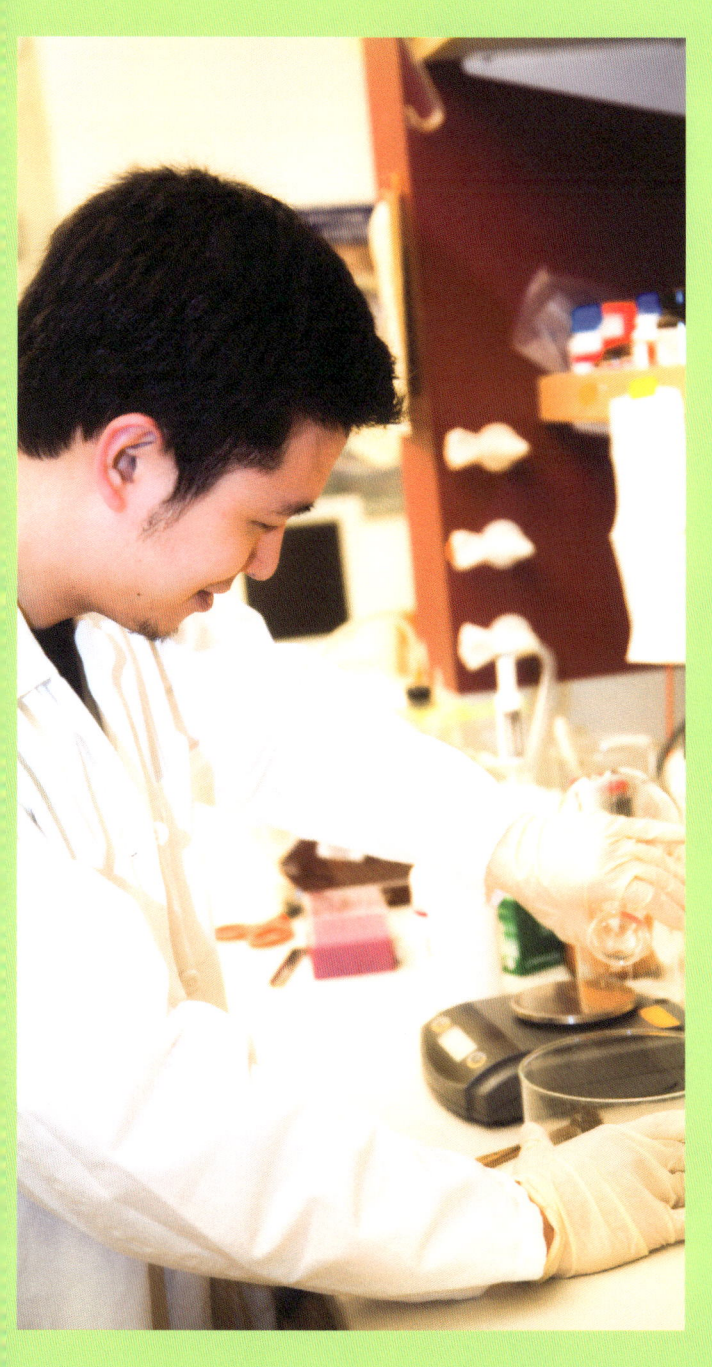

Some diseases, like the common cold, may never have a cure.

New treatments sometimes come about as a result of other, earlier discoveries, and sometimes by accident. Researchers then test these discoveries in laboratories and on sample patients.

Research takes lots of money. This means scientists tend to focus their time and attention on diseases that are the most serious and life-threatening. Research can be a long, slow process. But scientists are working hard to find the weapons to fight our tiniest enemies.

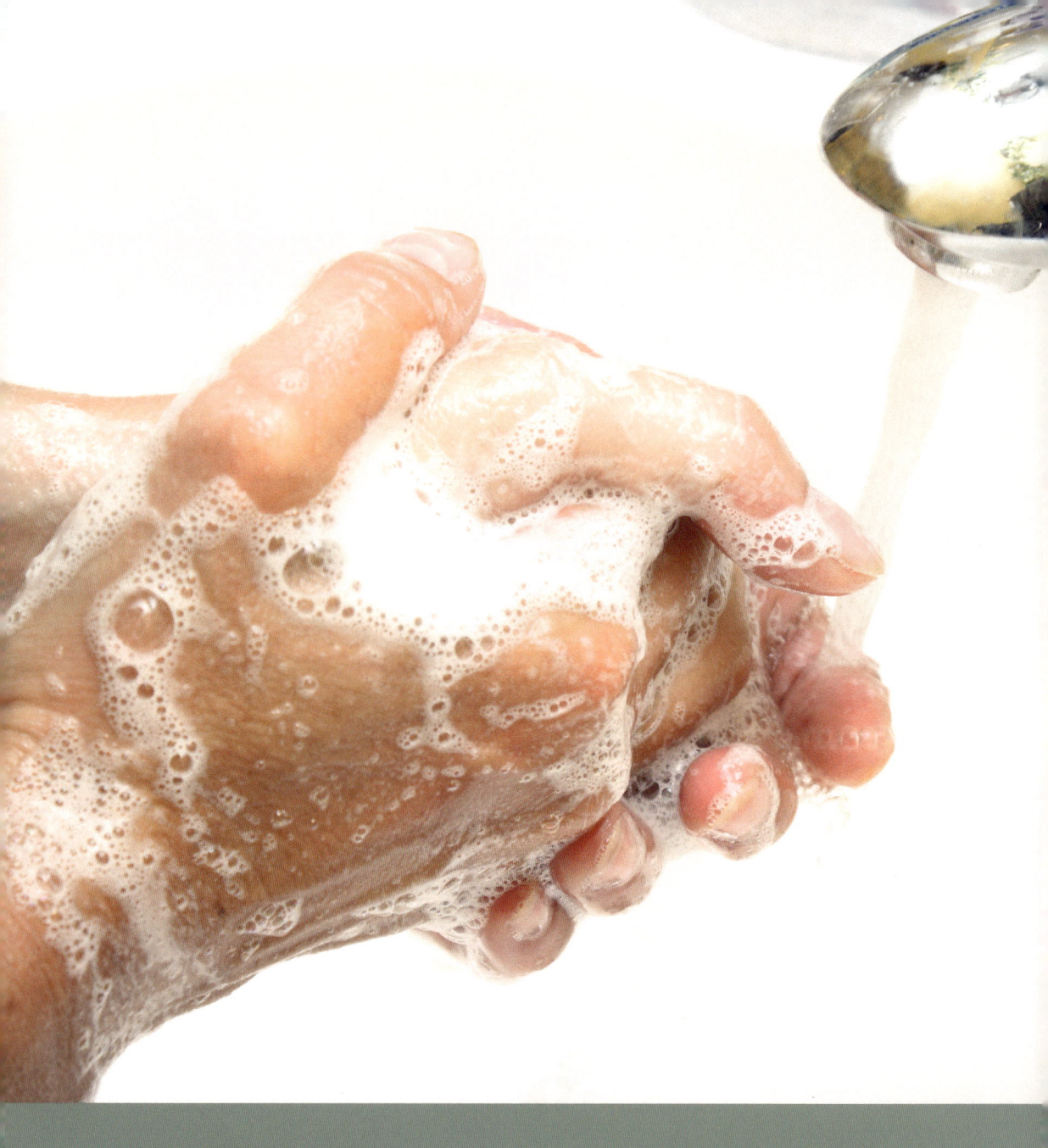

What Can You Do to Stay Healthy?

Did You Know?

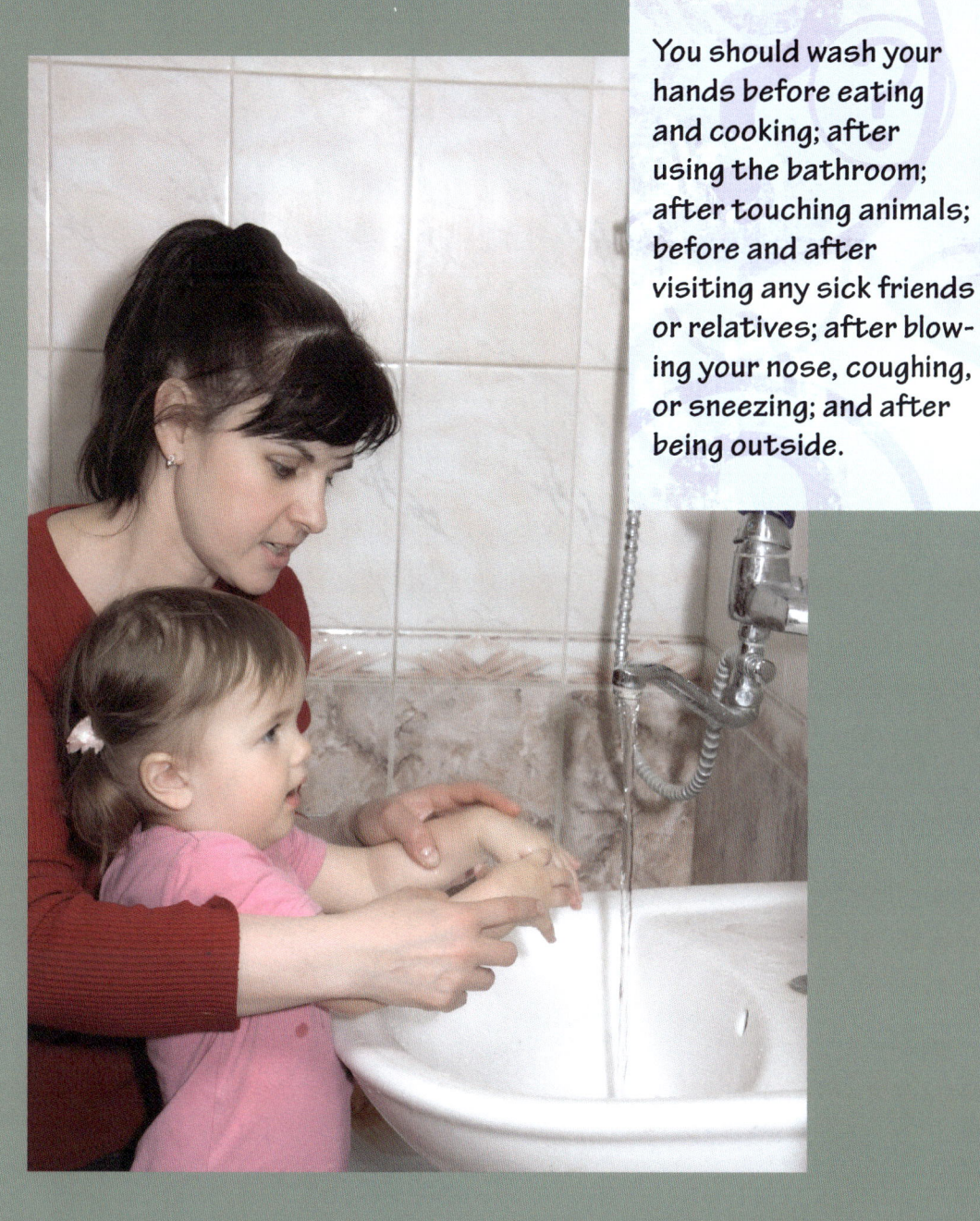

You should wash your hands before eating and cooking; after using the bathroom; after touching animals; before and after visiting any sick friends or relatives; after blowing your nose, coughing, or sneezing; and after being outside.

The best way to fight bacteria and viruses is very simple:

WASH YOUR HANDS!

Soap and warm water kill germs. And dead germs can't make you sick.

What Else Can You Do to Stay Healthy?

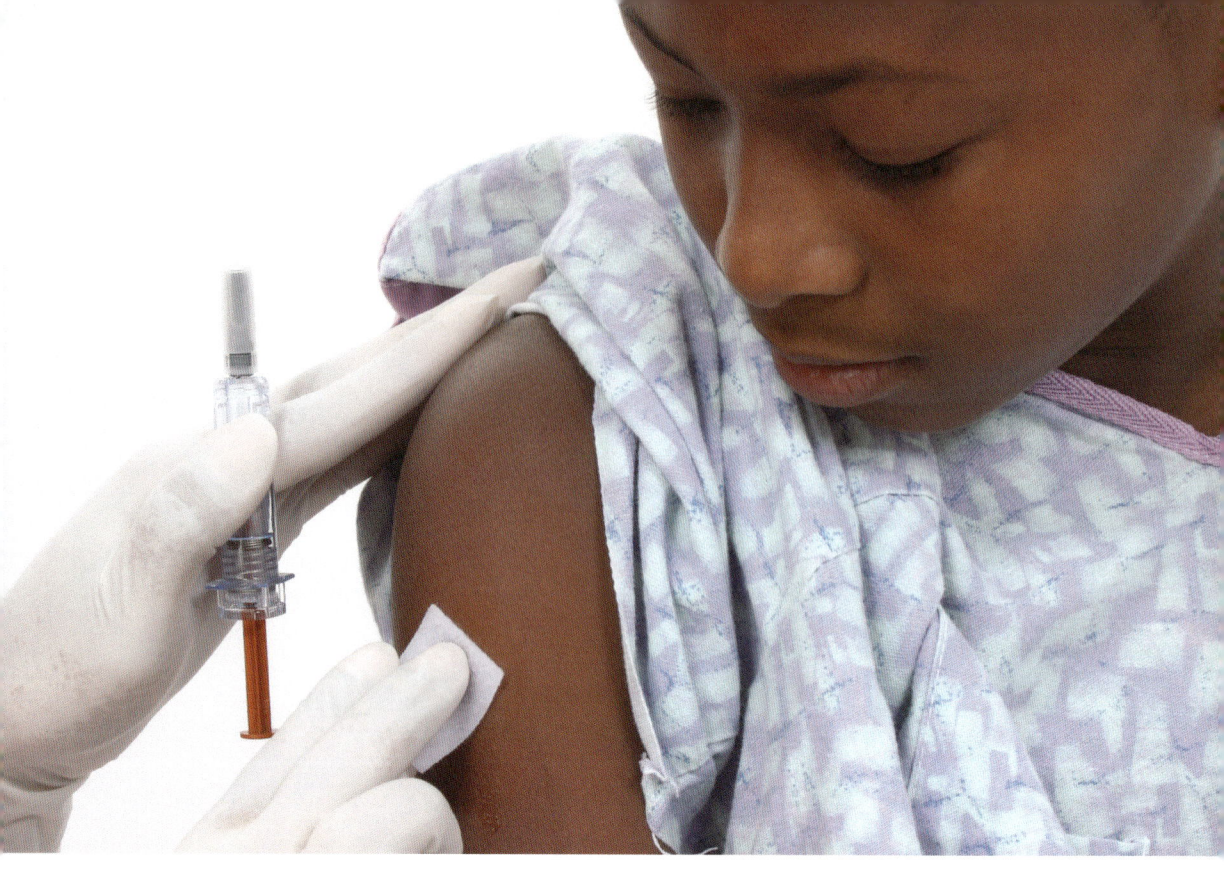

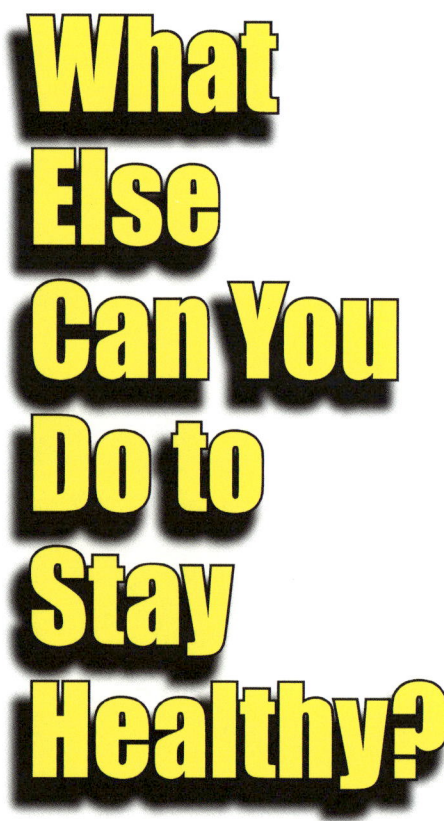

Stay healthy by getting the vaccinations (shots) you need. They may hurt, but a one-second needle prick is a lot better than getting sick!

Tired bodies that don't eat healthy foods have weaker immune systems. This means they're more likely to get sick. So get plenty of sleep and eat a healthy diet that includes fruit, vegetables, grains, and meat or other *protein*. If you do, you'll be better able to fight off your body's tiny enemies!

Words to Know

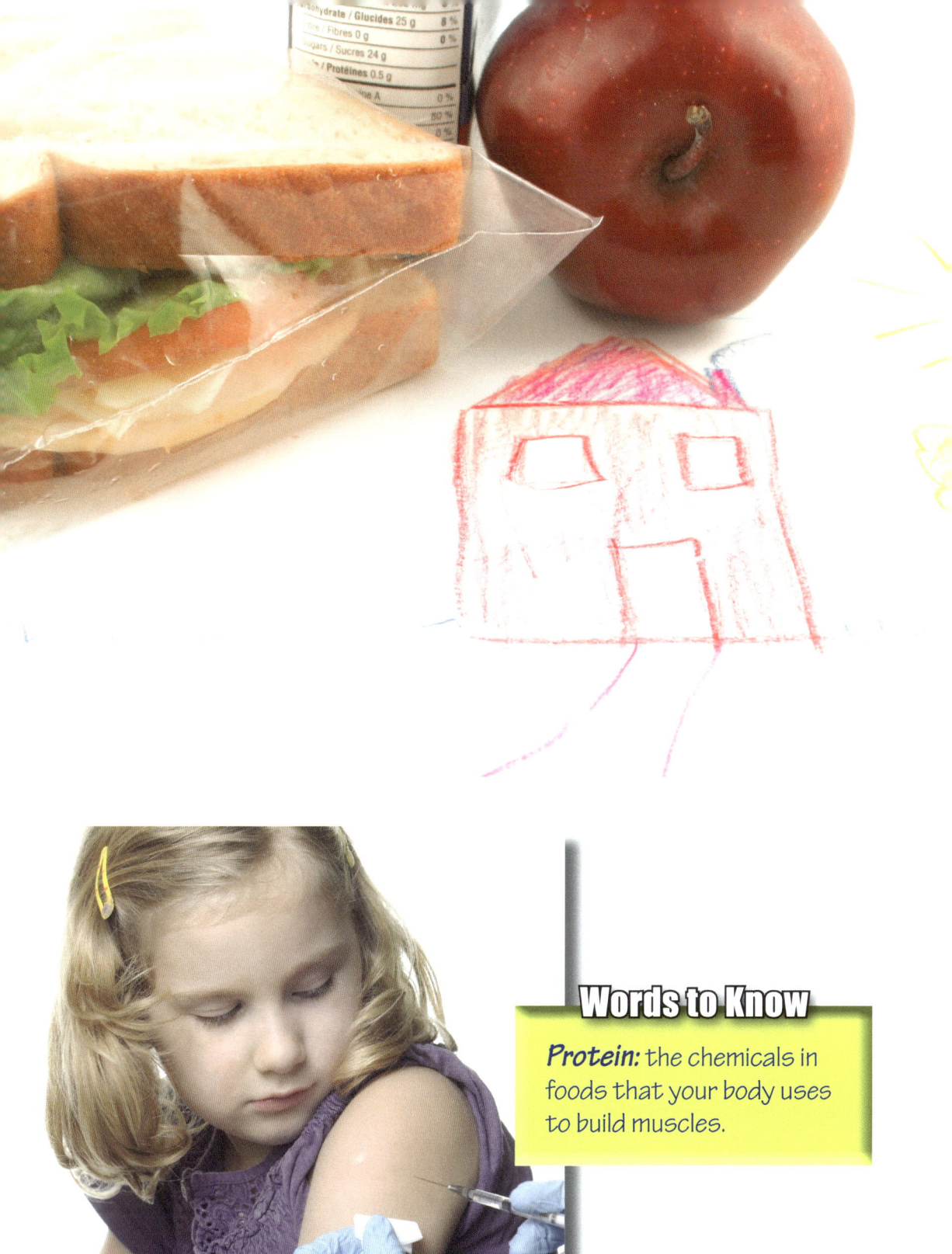

Protein: the chemicals in foods that your body uses to build muscles.

55

Real Kids

Eseko's family lived in the Darfur region of Sudan, until the Janjaweed militia came and attacked his village. Then, his family fled to Chad, where they now stay in a huge refugee camp. Water is scarce, and while people try their best, it is hard to keep things clean. First one of his friends and then his brother died of cholera. They caught this disease from drinking dirty water. Many other people in the camp were sick with cholera also. Things were very bad, but then the United Nations arrived to build toilets and wells. The UN also taught the people in the camp better ways to stay clean. Eseko and his family learned how to kill germs on their hands and foods. Now the camp is a healthier place. Eseko hopes that no one else he loves will die from cholera.

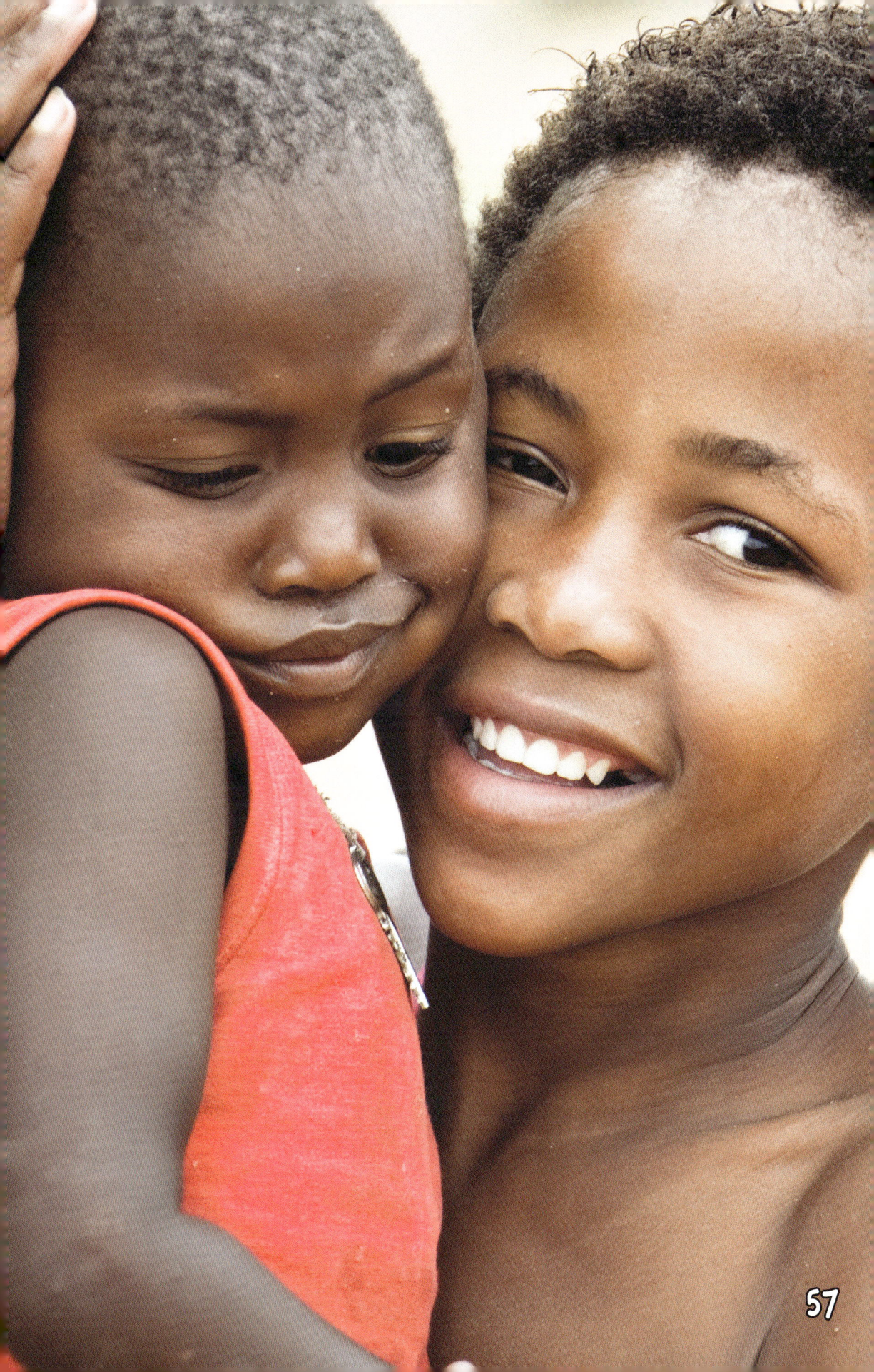

Real Kids

Bassira Saadou and her two siblings grew up being scared of the nighttime. They live in a city in Niger, where malaria is a common disease. Mosquitoes are most active around nightfall, so they tend to bite while people are asleep. Bassira's baby brother died from malaria.

But now, thanks to aid from the government of Niger, the Saadou children sleep under an insecticide-treated mosquito net. Thanks to this, Bassira has a far better chance of growing up healthy.

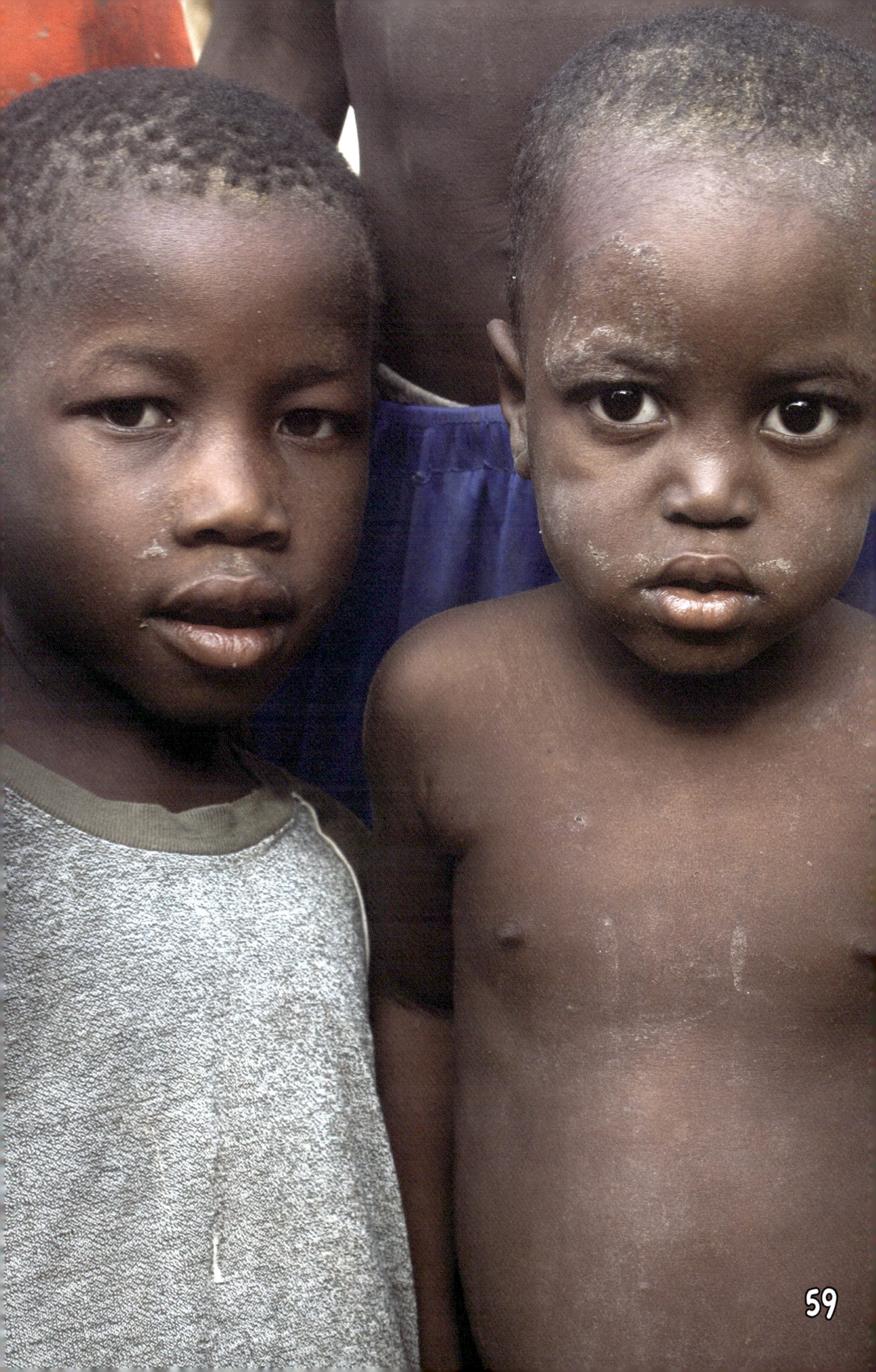

Find Out More

What Are Germs?
www.kidshealth.org/kid/talk/qa/germs.html

All About Viruses
www.livescience.com/topics/virus

E. Coli
kidshealth.org/kid/stay_healthy/food/ecoli.html

Herpes
herpes-coldsores.com

HIV and AIDS
www.kidshealth.org/kid/health_problems/infection/hiv.html

Influenza
www.medicinenet.com/influenza/article.htm

MRSA
www.mayoclinic.com/health/mrsa/DS00735

Rhinovirus (common cold)
www.webmd.com/cold-and-flu/cold-guide/common_cold_causes

Staph Infections
www.kidshealth.org/teen/infections/bacterial_viral/staph.html

Streptococcal Infections
www.nlm.nih.gov/medlineplus/streptococcalinfections.html

What Are Bacteria?
archive.food.gov.uk/hea/711/english/part1.html

Index

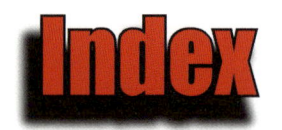

anthrax 26–27
antibiotics 7, 28–31

bacteria 7, 9, 12–26, 28–32, 50, 53

common cold 36–37, 39, 41, 51, 61
cough 24, 36–38, 48, 53

DNA 31

E. coli 7, 22–23

fever 19–20, 35–36, 41, 43, 45

germs 7–11, 18, 21, 29, 31, 34, 50, 53, 56

herpes 7, 42
HIV 7, 46, 48, 50

immune system 34–35, 46–47, 54
influenza (flu) 7, 19, 27, 40–41, 46, 48–49
intestines 22–23, 26

lungs 19, 21, 24–26, 36

microbes 9
mouth 13, 21

pinkeye 38–39
pneumonia 20–21

rhinovirus 37

saliva 7, 10
skin 7, 8, 10, 17, 19–20, 25–26
soil 12–13
staph infection 16–19
stomach 17, 20, 22, 23, 26
strep infection 20

throat 17, 20–21, 36
toxins 15, 22
tuberculosis (TB) 7, 24–25

vaccines 7, 49–50
viruses 7, 9, 32–37, 42, 48–49, 53

water 7, 11–13, 23, 38, 53, 56
West Nile virus 44–45

Picture Credits

Dreamstime.com:
  8: Alexstar
  9: Clearviewstock
  10: Rafael Angel Irusta Machin
  11: Kirsty Pargeter
  12-13: Bram Janssens
  14 (background): Eti Swinford
  14 (top): Tmorris9
  14 (middle): Rajcreationzs
  14 (bottom): José Marafona
  15: Suzanne Tucker
  19: Sebastian Kaulitzki
  20: Sebastian Kaulitzki
  21: Cheryl Casey
  22: Sebastian Kaulitzki
  23: Richard Wozniak
  26 (top): Leigh Prather
  26 (bottom): Carolina K. Smith M.d.
  27: Dtfoxfoto
  28 (top): Olha Rohulya
  28 (bottom): Bialasiewicz
  29: Monika Wisniewska
  30: Sebastian Kaulitzki
  31: Billyfoto
  32: Pseudolongino
  33: Alila07
  34: Glenda Powers
  35: Sebastian Kaulitzki
  36: Fred Goldstein
  37: Pirus01
  38: Crystal Craig
  39 left: Photographerlondon
  39 right: Pavel Losevsky
  41 top: Sparkia
  41 bottom: Thomas Perkins
  42: Apichsn
  44 top: Photoroller
  44 bottom: Nathalie Speliers Ufermann
  45 bottom: Anton Harder
  48: Putilich
  49: Showface
  50: Ggw1962
  51: Suprijono Suharjoto
  52: Matthew Benoit
  53: Annaigonina908
  54: Photoeuphoria
  55 top: Gvictoria
  55 bottom: Itsmejust
  57: Lucian Coman
  59: Aprescindere

www.cdc.gov:
  43: Centers for Disease Control
  45 top: Centers for Disease Control
  45 middle: Centers for Disease Control

nih.gov:
  18: National Institute of Health
  24 (bottom): National Institutes of Health

phil.cdc.gov:
  16: Public Health Image Library
  24 (top): Public Health Image Library
  25: Public Health Image Library
  40: CDC Public Health Image Library
  46: CDC Public Health Image Library
  47: CDC Public Health Image Library

To the best knowledge of the publisher, all other images are in the public domain. If any image has been inadvertently uncredited, please notify Village Earth Press, Vestal, New York 13850, so that rectification can be made for future printings.

About the Author

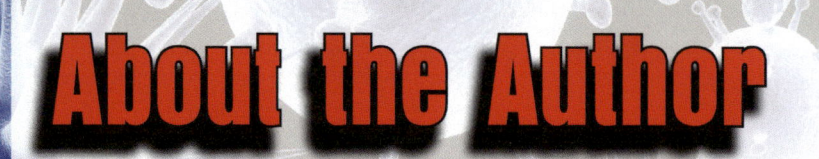

Rae Simons has written many books for young adults and children. She lives with her family in New York State in the United States.

About the Consultant

Elise DeVore Berlan, MD, MPH, FAAP, is a faculty member of the Division of Adolescent Health at Nationwide Children's Hospital and an Assistant Professor of Clinical Pediatrics at the Ohio State University College of Medicine. She completed her fellowship in adolescent medicine at Children's Hospital Boston and obtained a master's degree in public health at the Harvard School of Public Health. Dr. Berlan completed her residency in pediatrics at the Children's Hospital of Philadelphia, where she also served an additional year as chief resident. She received her medical degree from the University of Iowa College of Medicine.